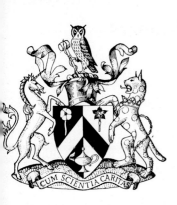

Significant Event Auditing

A Study of the Feasibility and Potential of Case-based Auditing in Primary Medical Care

MICHAEL PRINGLE MD, FRCGP
Department of General Practice
University of Nottingham

COLIN P BRADLEY MD, FRCGP
Department of General Practice
University of Birmingham

CATHERINE M CARMICHAEL BMedSci (Hons), MB BCh, MSc
United Health
Scunthorpe and Grimsby Health Authority

HEATHER WALLIS SRN
ANNE MOORE BSc (Hons)
Department of General Practice
University of Nottingham

Published by
The Royal College of General Practitioners

March 1995

The Royal College of General Practitioners

Charter

The Royal College of General Practitioners was founded in 1952, with this object:

"To encourage, foster, and maintain the highest possible standards in general medical practice and for that purpose to take or join with others in taking steps consistent with the charitable nature of that object which may assist towards the same."

Among its responsibilities under its Royal Charter the College is entitled to:

"Encourage the publication by general medical practitioners of research into medical or scientific subjects with a view to the improvement of general medical practice in any field and to undertake or assist others in undertaking such research.

"Diffuse information on all matters affecting general medical practice and establish, print, publish, issue and circulate such papers, journals, magazines, books, periodicals, and publications and hold such meetings, conferences, seminars, and instructional courses as may assist the object of the College."

College Headquarters

The headquarters of the Royal College is at 14 Princes Gate, Hyde Park, London SW7 1PU (Telephone: 0171-581 3232). Enquiries should be addressed to the General Manager.

Exeter Publications Office

The Publications Office publishes on behalf of the College the series of *Policy Statements, Reports from General Practice, Occasional Papers*, and books and booklets. It also co-ordinates material for the *RCGP Members' Reference Book*. Enquiries are welcomed and should be addressed to the Honorary Editor, 9 Marlborough Road, Exeter, Devon EX2 4TJ (Telephone: 01392 57938).

Occasional Papers

The *Occasional Paper* series was established in 1976 to offer authors the opportunity to publish manuscripts too long for publication as articles and too short for books. They are assessed for academic acceptability by members of the Editorial Board and other professionals with special interests. Readers should note that they express the views of the authors, and not the College, unless otherwise stated.

Copyright

Contents

Editor's Preface

T HE BIGGEST single topic among the *Occasional Papers* has been education in relation to the discipline of general practice. The latest *Occasional Paper*, number 70, continues this theme placing emphasis on education through audit or assessment, and offering new evidence of the importance of significant event auditing in the context of general practice.

The idea of following up an important event in an organization is not, of course, new. 'Critical incident analysis' was the term in vogue in the 1970s, particularly in North America, and it was normal practice in many walks of life to use this method of review. For example, when training pilots and crew in aircraft safety it was—and still is—common practice to examine difficult incidents, notably 'near-misses', and review them with particular reference to identifying lessons to be learnt for the future. (It is important to note, however, that the authors of this *Occasional Paper* have deliberately chosen the term 'significant' event auditing as regularly they point out that notable events can be a cause for celebration as well as regret.)

The emphasis in medical audit in general practice over the last twenty years has been very much on the group, particularly in relation to sets of patients with common conditions, such as asthma, diabetes and hypertension. The importance of this new *Occasional Paper* is that it provides an alternative approach which focuses on a particular incident or episode and usually on a particular patient. Professor Pringle and his colleagues explain how this heightens the emotional significance of the incident and enables a wider range of issues, including personal, clinical, psychological and social factors, to be taken into account. Throughout their paper they make a powerful case for examining such issues but they go further than any authors before them in that they not only report a survey of the use of this method, but at the same time report a survey of doctors undertaking conventional audit and then seek to tease out comparisons between the two methods. They rightly and cautiously say that whilst making the case for the new method they want to make it clear that conventional audit using groups and predetermined criteria remains valid and needs to continue in general practice.

The importance of this development thus lies in its broadening, not narrowing, of audit methods. Significant event auditing is not an alternative to conventional audit but an extension of it, and moreover it is a technique which is very much in tune with current educational thinking in general practice because its characteristics—rigorous discussion, emphasis on individual patients, and so on—belong to qualitative analysis rather than the quantitative methods which have been predominant in the last two decades.

Balint's work is an important early example of qualitative research, as it also depended on a group, but—a pointer for the future—it was a group not of general practitioners from different practices but of doctors and often their team colleagues within a single practice.

Pringle and his colleagues have taken this one step further. They can be seen as helping to define the boundary between, for example, the disciplines of public health medicine, which centres on groups of the population, and general practice, which is ultimately a personal and clinical discipline for medical generalists; their work may yet prove to mark the swing of a pendulum away from the public health approach, which has dominated audit thinking for the last generation, towards a greater emphasis on the highly personal and specific issues of caring for individual people, in particular homes and families, at a particular point in time. Indeed it highlights, as few other methods have done, the College motto, *Cum scientia caritas* ("compassion with science"), which so cleverly reflects the recurring theme of the interplay between personal factors and scientific factors in the discipline of general practice.

This *Occasional Paper* signals a new direction of thinking about audit in three quite different ways: it places a new emphasis on qualitative review as opposed to quantitative methods; it places a new emphasis on the whole person taking physical, psychological and social factors into account; and it places a new emphasis on people working together in the practice setting rather than elsewhere.

We commend this paper to our readers and look forward to further developments in this field.

DENIS PEREIRA GRAY
Honorary Editor
College Publications

9 Marlborough Road
Exeter EX2 4TJ

January 1995

Preface

M Y PRACTICE began to audit in the mid-1980s. The first steps were tentative and crude; there were no protocols, no standards, and no completed audit cycles. It was just a case of "look and see". By 1989 three of us were ready for the challenge of Fellowship by Assessment and this proved to be one of two seminal events in our quality culture.

Fellowship by Assessment gave us the motivation to draw up a basic range of clinical and managerial protocols and to evaluate our care critically against agreed standards. In doing so we became painfully aware that there is a world of difference between agreeing a standard and living up to it in day-to-day clinical care.

About three months after our success in Fellowship by Assessment I was surprised to see "Clinical audit" as an agenda item for a practice meeting. I felt that we had demonstrated our commitment and that no more was required. My partner, however, introduced the item with words that struck home to us all: "We may have satisfied them, but have we satisfied ourselves? We have met their standards but we know we can do better than that."

His thesis, to which I readily subscribed, was that drawing up protocols and standards, and then measuring our care against them, was the easy, mechanistic part. The challenge was to keep improving—and that required a continuing commitment to change. From that meeting onwards we embarked on a programme of protocol review, regular auditing and the publication of our results.

It might be thought that this history should engender a warm glow of self-satisfaction. Clearly our practice is determined to deliver quality of care in reality, not just by paying lip service. There is, however, a negative aspect—the process started to become sterile. We chased our recording of the smoking habits of patients with diabetes from under 10% to over 90%, but is that real quality, or just an illusion based on better recording habits? Were we really helping those diabetics who smoked to give up?

It was in this climate of self-doubt that the second key event occurred—one which had profound implications for our quality culture. A patient died.

I was sitting in my room, halfway through evening surgery, when there was a knock on the door. I apologized to my patient and ran to the treatment room where a man of 58 had had a cardiac arrest. Despite three doctors being in attendance, despite a high level of equipment, the patient died. That night we slunk home to our families aware that we had been challenged and found wanting.

Every practice has similar tales; every practitioner experiences the devastation of losing a battle that might have been won. But most practices console themselves and carry on—indeed that would have been our normal practice. On this occasion we responded in a new way. We called a meeting.

The discussion was painful and emotional. We were, however, determined to ensure that all the lessons for quality were learnt. The first decision was a relatively easy one: our resuscitation might have been successful if we had had a defibrillator. We were overwhelmed by the community response and the funds for a defibrillator were raised within a month.

The more difficult discussions centred around our own clinical competence and the equipment that we had available to us. We realized that it was, for most of us, many years since we had been called on to do a full-scale resuscitation and we were, frankly, rusty. A programme of regular instruction and refreshing of emergency skills has been put in place and continues to this day.

The equipment in the medical centre is now checked regularly and the drugs for acute care are kept in a special tray, clearly labelled, which can be taken to the site of an emergency in the building. The drugs that we carry in our cars were reviewed and are regularly maintained by a designated member of staff.

One event—admittedly an exceedingly traumatic one—led to a chain reaction of desirable changes. This was our baptism of fire in significant event auditing. To this day we continue to hold meetings every month at which we discuss key events in the life of the practice, clinical and administrative, and try to learn the lessons from them. We still do traditional audits, of course, but we have added a new dimension.

Our experience suggests that traditional audits appeal to the intellect. There is no disputing, for example, that only one in three patients with hypertension has a urea level recorded within the past year, and there is no disputing the need to improve. However, change is an emotional process and we all find it difficult to link intellectual decisions into change.

Significant event auditing, on the other hand, is less intellectually rigorous; a practice can spend an hour discussing an event which is unlikely ever to recur in the working lives of members of the team. It has, however, a strong emotional content which makes a link into change of behaviour much more powerful.

The challenge seems to be, therefore, to harness both forms of medical audit into a coherent culture where, for example, a conventional audit showing a low level of urea recording in patients with hypertension is reinforced by discussion of a patient who went into renal failure; a conventional audit of the smoking habits of patients is reinforced by discussion of a patient diagnosed with carcinoma of the bronchus; or an audit of appointment availability is linked to a patient who complains of having to wait too long to see a doctor.

Moreover, the semantics are important. We do not talk of 'critical incident analysis' because we often celebrate our care; we do not like the quasi-judicial intonations of 'incident'; and our discussions are more qualitative than the word 'analysis' might suggest. We have found that 'significant event auditing' exactly matches what we feel about the process.

Having had a conversion on the road to quality, having learnt to appreciate a new concept in the development of a quality culture, I discovered that I was far from alone. Colin Bradley had been talking about significant events for months, and we agreed to join forces in putting together a research protocol. Here, some four years later, is the result. Without Department of Health funding and the co-operation of twenty practices throughout Lincolnshire and Manchester it would not have been possible. But without the death of a man in the treatment room of my medical centre it would not have been conceived.

MIKE PRINGLE
February 1994

Significant Event Auditing

A Study of the Feasibility and Potential of Case-based Auditing in Primary Medical Care

INTRODUCTION

THE IDEA of reviewing the quality of medical care with a view to its improvement is certainly not a new one. The Code of Hamurabi (Babylonian king, 1728–1686 BC), which stipulated that doctors whose treatments failed should have their hands cut off, is often quoted as the earliest example of medical audit (Baker, 1993). Though the remedy for dealing with deficiencies in care was rather draconian, performance was assessed on a case-by-case basis beginning with an evaluation of the outcome. This has been the basis of many later, highly successful applications of the principle of performance review.

Case review is one of the oldest principles underlying the development of medicine. It has been used by some of the greatest doyens of medicine, such as Osler and Sydenham, to advance understanding of health and disease, and they have been notable for their meticulous review of the outcomes of single cases. Similar close observation of psychopathology by Freud has given birth to a whole specialism within psychiatry. But just as single case review was used to learn about disease, and the principles of its management and understanding of disease was put on a firmer scientific footing, and just as management could be defined more systematically, the principle of case review has come to be used rather more to ensure that existing knowledge is being properly applied. Thus, one can see the essence of this approach being applied in the case of confidential enquiries into maternal deaths (DHSS, 1986), enquiries into anaesthetic deaths (Lunn and Musher, 1982), deaths in people under 50 years (Medical Services, 1978), the National Confidential Enquiry into peri-operative deaths (Buck et al., 1987), and in the pioneering work of Codman (1916) in the US. The same philosophy of structured review of single cases with a view to learning for the future is also the basis of the traditional grand round or clinico-pathological conference and is also an underlying principle of postmortems. The principles have also been extended into psychiatry and have given rise to the notion of the psychological postmortem (Barrowclough et al., 1974). The essential points are that performance is reviewed systematically following an undesirable outcome with a view to discovering features of the case that may have contributed to that outcome and then modifying procedures or practices to avoid their future recurrence.

An alternative model for the assessment of the quality of medical care uses a quantitative approach based on observations of a large number of patients regarding the presence or absence of certain features of their care thought to be associated with good medical practice. An early example of this more statistical approach was demonstrated by Florence Nightingale when she collected mortality and morbidity statistics on soldiers in the Crimean War and related these to features of their medical and nursing care (Baly, 1986). This approach also underlies the work of Donabedian, who was a major influence on the development of medical audit in general practice in the United Kingdom (Donabedian, 1982; Pendleton et al., 1986). Thus early examples of audit in general practice in the United Kingdom were clearly based on a method of audit that involved collection of data on parameters or markers of care (most usually the process of care), comparison with a (usually pre-specified) standard, and had a longer-term view of repeating the process cyclically as described in the "audit cycle" (Shaw, 1980).

This approach was further encouraged by the development of practice activity analysis (PAA) by the RCGP Birmingham Research Unit, which put the data collection and analytical tools for the task of cohort-based audit into the hands of general practitioners (Crombie and Fleming, 1988). The entire concept of audit was given a further boost by the College's Quality Initiative (RCGP, 1985a) and was enshrined in the government's expectation of professional performance in the NHS reforms (DoH, 1989). Of all the health service reforms imposed by the United Kingdom government in 1990, it is the one which had and continues to have the broadest support of the profession as represented by organizations such as the Royal College of General Practitioners and British Medical Association. It now has its own clearly identified funding and infrastructure in the form of medical audit advisory groups (MAAGs) (DoH, 1990). While all this is welcome, the official sanction and support has been built around a fairly narrow conception of what constitutes audit. The quantitative model clearly predominates in the thinking of the government and others, and more qualitative approaches were explicitly discouraged by the Standing Medical Advisory Committee's interdict that "the 'grand round' or 'interesting case' type of meeting does not meet the requirements of medical audit" (SMAC, 1990).

This is not to say that other forms of performance review are not going on in parallel. Informal review of cases is part of the medical culture and occurs over coffee or in the reception area in all practices. It has also been incorporated in a more formal way into general practitioner training in the form of random case analysis and problem case analysis (Buckley, 1990). The work of Balint groups, while clearly focused on achieving psychotherapeutic goals for both doctor and patient, by virtue of their method includes an element of performance evaluation (Balint, 1964). The "What Sort of Doctor?" initiative (RCGP, 1985b) clearly promotes a form of performance review which includes individual case-by-case assessment of performance and this idea is being carried forward within the procedure for obtaining Fellowship by Assessment (RCGP, 1990). Furthermore, some key figures in the promotion of quality assurance in general practice are broadly supportive of the case-based approach, though they have either not specified a methodology or have described a methodology that remains untested (Buckley, 1990; Hughes and Humphreys, 1990; Irvine, 1990; Marinker, 1990). Bradley (1992) has identified some of the potential sources of the reservations about relying on single cases or instances and has proposed the application of the principles of critical incident technique to overcome these difficulties. This gives rise to a form of medical audit known as 'significant event analysis'.

In significant event analysis, individual cases in which there has been a significant occurrence (not necessarily involving an undesirable outcome for the patient) are analysed in a systematic and detailed way to ascertain what can be learnt about the overall quality of care and to indicate changes that might lead to future improvements. Significant events, because they are de facto emotionally charged and compel one to take stock, may be powerful motivators to change behaviour providing that the potential for them to provoke a barrier of defensiveness is recognized and overcome. A more formalized analysis endeavours to ensure that such opportunities for self-examination are properly exploited and not covered up while seeking to avoid excessive responses or inappropriate changes. The procedure involves the selection and collection of suitable events for analysis followed by meetings to discuss how practice or procedure might be modified to avoid undesirable outcomes in the future. These are later followed by a further review of performance to see if the modifications have been made and if they have achieved their objective.

The technique has much in common with the idea of occurrence screening (Bennett and Walshe, 1990) inasmuch as it is concerned with retrospective review of individual cases but differs from this in that it is not so exclusively concerned with fault finding and the limiting of exposure to medico–legal risk; it is as open to the possibility of affirming good practice as it is to identifying deficiencies and gaps in care and it seeks to involve the whole team in remedying the situation. The retrospective review of individual cases is also a feature of the confidential enquiry approach adopted in hospital practice and applied to obstetric care and surgery (Lunn and Musher, 1982; Buck et al., 1987). However, because of their confidential nature, these give feedback that is non-specific. This approach, which involves seeking avoidable and unavoidable causes, is rather too close to the blame attribution culture still quite prevalent in hospital case conferences. Seeking to attach blame to individuals in the more direct and personalized feedback involved in significant event analysis runs counter to the prevailing general practice culture and would be unhelpful and demoralizing. Hence it must be avoided. Significant event analysis draws rather more on the philosophy of critical incident technique (Flanagan, 1954; Bradley, 1992) or on what has come to be known in general practice teaching as the Pendleton approach, in which both positive and negative aspects of behaviour are considered (Pendleton et al., 1984). Positive achievements are acknowledged and rewarded as a necessary prerequisite to a constructive approach to the examination of perceived deficiencies.

Contrasting approaches to performance review

Thus, it may be seen that there are two contrasting approaches to performance review available to general practitioners. The first we have chosen to call the conventional approach. This refers to the now well described cyclical process consisting of choosing an area of medical practice to be evaluated, defining standards for performance in that area, measuring actual performance against that standard, deciding on changes needed to bring performance closer to the standard, implementing the changes and then, after an interval, reviewing performance against the standards to ensure that the desired improvement has occurred.

Significant event auditing can also be described as a multi-stage procedure. Events deemed to be significant, which include certain deaths, emergencies, and clinical and administrative events, are selected for consideration. A mechanism is then set up to identify such events. Meetings of the team are arranged for the events to be discussed and analysed. On the basis of a structured discussion decisions are made to seek to improve the quality of care for the future. An agreement is also made for the future review of performance in respect of the same problem and this review may well consist of a conventional audit.

Conventional audit involves the systematic analysis of predetermined data, usually of a quantitative nature, regarding the care of a cohort of patients usually sharing a single problem. There is an assumption that the available data are a reliable reflection of the reality of the care delivered, though it is recognized that such data may not always be accurate and are often incomplete, especially in respect of important negative findings. The process is tightly structured and involves a largely cerebral process not usually requiring a great deal of emotional involvement.

By contrast, significant event analysis is a rather less rigidly restricted review of any and all information, including quite subjective judgements, about the care of single patients. Records are used but opinion and impressions are also valued in the case review. Significant event analysis is less tightly structured, although it can be just as rigorous. It allows for, indeed encourages, emotional involvement. It focuses, at least initially, on outcomes but reviews processes too.

SIGNIFICANT EVENT AUDITING

Appendix 1 sets out a short user's guide to significant event auditing, which readers may find helpful; the following section describes in greater detail the steps to be taken.

Steps to be taken

The steps to be taken in the analysis of a significant event are as follows:

1. Consider the events to be audited
2. Collect data on these events
3. Hold a meeting to discuss the events. The meeting could cover some or all of the following points:

   - immediate management of the case
   - preventive care opportunities
   - follow-up of the case

- implications for the family/community
- interface issues
- team issues
- action to be taken/policy decisions to be made
- follow-up arrangements

4. Documentation.

1. Consideration of significant events for audit

Any event thought by anyone in the team to be significant in the care of patients or the conduct of the practice should be open for consideration. However, practices are advised to give some consideration to the events they would want to analyse before starting to use this method of audit. A good idea is to begin with a core list (such as that given on page 6) and to refine this according to local needs and interests. This can be done at a meeting of the primary health care team. Some very common events, while undoubtedly significant in some respects, may fail to stimulate much interest or provoke much discussion, and their analysis will quickly lead to apathy and perhaps disillusionment with the method. On the other hand, one should not rely only on events of indisputable significance that occur too infrequently, as they will fail to generate sufficient material for analysis and again the method will fall into disuse.

Having a list serves mainly as an *aide mémoire* to doctors and other staff to encourage the collection of suitable events for subsequent discussion and analysis. Although one may start with an existing list (page 6), practices are strongly encouraged to adapt and modify it, or to agree an alternative list of their own. Appendices 2, 3 and 4 of this document will give readers some further ideas of possible events to be considered based on those generated by participants in this study.

2. Data collection

(a) Identification of events for analysis

Having agreed a list, one needs to set up mechanisms within the practice to ensure the listed events are spotted. For instance, it is usually a good idea to establish a method for scanning incoming and outgoing post for significant events occurring to patients who have contact with agencies outside the practice. Other methods that have been tried include placing encounter forms on the doctors' desks and reminders at regular intervals in their intrays or pigeon-holes. Where the practice is recording all encounters on computer this may be used to search for suitable events.

(b) Recording details of cases

In order to analyse an event it is important to examine the existing patient record even though much material vital to understanding the significance of the event will reside largely in people's heads. It is also a good idea, if possible, to have some means of recording a few details, however brief, when the event first comes to attention. A pre-designed form to extract pertinent details from the record (and indeed from team members' recollections) may also be employed to gain more details prior to the meeting. In a case of myocardial infarction, for instance, one would examine the record for details of immediate care; past medical history especially of relevant conditions such as diabetes; and for evidence of health promotion especially in respect of smoking and alcohol. In addition, the record needs to be scrutinized for details of drug therapy and for evidence pertaining to any contact with hospital(s) such as letters and discharge summaries. If such a pre-designed form is used, a decision may have to be made about how far back in the record one should go when extracting details. However, such a decision should not be allowed to preclude consideration of events further back in the history if these are thought to have some bearing at the time of the meeting. Prior consideration of what material to collect for the meeting also provides an opportunity of obtaining relevant scientific papers or articles to inform the discussion. This was an opportunity exploited by several of our study practices.

3. Significant events meetings

(a) Implications of events

The central component of significant event auditing is the meeting held to discuss events. Beyond discussing what happened and why, a key function of the meeting is to consider the implications of the event for the quality of care given to patients generally and to make policy decisions aimed at improving the quality of care. These meetings should be held at a pre-arranged time and place; they should be chaired; they should lead to firm decisions about how care might be improved; and these decisions should be recorded for later review.

Once significant event auditing is up and running, meetings should begin with a review of any outstanding matters regarding previously analysed cases. In particular, this is a valuable opportunity to ensure that decisions made at previous meetings have been followed up. Then the list of cases for possible analysis at that meeting is perused. Participants may be invited to select cases from those with which they were involved. Alternatively, all participants may be asked to pick cases they would like to hear about. Very occasionally an event may be deemed too sensitive or its discussion be too emotionally charged for one or more participants, and everyone should have a right of veto of the analysis of such events. However, it is important that the exercise of this right is confined to the most exceptional circumstances and people should be encouraged gently not to hide too often behind its shield. While the right of veto is an important safeguard of people's sensibilities and dignity, its abuse could significantly diminish the power of this potentially most incisive form of critical self-appraisal.

(b) Discussion of cases

Discussion of each case selected for analysis is led by the person(s) who are/were primarily involved in the care of the patient, or in the matter to be discussed if it is a largely administrative issue. Everyone closely involved in the case should be encouraged to comment on aspects of the case where quality was of a demonstrably high standard. Then everyone should be encouraged to suggest ways of making improvements that would address any deficiencies in care that have been exposed. While practices should feel free to conduct meetings as they see fit, a suggested agenda for the meeting is offered below (Figure 1). Practices should judge for themselves how many such issues ought to be, or indeed can be, considered in respect of any significant event.

(c) Decisions about cases

A key feature of this form of case discussion is that it leads to decisions being made for each case. Four types of decisions can be reached following significant event analysis. These are:

- that no change in current practice or procedures is required
- congratulations are deserved by the team
- a conventional cohort type audit is needed
- an immediate change to policies, practices or procedures is required and will be implemented.

(d) Follow-up

Clearly, if significant event analysis is to fit within the audit model there must also be some follow-up. What follow-up is done and how it is done will very much depend on the conclusions and policy decisions of the significant events meeting. Occasionally, it may be decided that the best way to follow up the implementation of a new policy initiative is to continue to monitor the same types of events and to conduct further significant event analyses if and when another event occurs. The experience of people who have used significant event analysis, however, has been that the follow-up of a significant event is often best done by more conventional audit techniques. Because of this it may be seen that significant event analysis is a useful means of introducing audit and audit methods to a practice, though the demands on group working skills should not be underestimated. Few doctors can resist the opportunity to discuss the case where something significant happened. Having highlighted problems and resolved to solve them, the importance and relevance of audit of one's work in the more conventional fashion becomes much clearer.

4. Documentation

It is important that significant event meetings and particularly decisions made during them are adequately documented. It is best to assign the role of record-keeper to someone at the meeting. That person should record brief notes on: the nature of the problem perceived; why it was deemed significant; aspects of care or running of the practice considered; implications for the team or other carers considered; and the decisions made. The record should also contain a clear statement regarding all commitments to action and the plans for future follow-up.

Figure 1   Suggested agenda for a significant event meeting

1. Review of previous meeting(s) and decisions

2. Case presentations

Concentrate on the facts of the case to begin with, keeping questions and interruptions to points of clarification. Then look at details of each case under whichever headings are appropriate:

(a) *Review of acute care/immediate problems*
- positive aspects of care
- aspects needing improvement

(b) *Review of possibilities for prevention*
- positive aspects of preventive care
- aspects needing improvement

(c) *Plan of action and follow-up*
- positive aspects of case
- aspects needing improvement

(d) *Implications for family/community (if any)*

(e) *Interface issues (if any)*

(f) *Team issues (if any)*

(g) *Summary*

(h) *Recommendations*
- These should reflect changes in policy or procedures designed to remedy any deficiencies in the quality of care exposed by the audit

3. Record key issues in minutes of the meeting

4. Date and time of next meeting

AIMS

Clearly, the authors of this study believe that significant event analysis has something to offer in the evaluation and improvement of the quality of care in general practice. However, given the widespread reservation about this approach and the unfamiliarity of general practice with such qualitative methods we set up a study with the following aims:

1. To explore the feasibility and acceptability of significant event auditing in a variety of general practice settings

2. To record the experience and reactions of practices carrying out conventional and case-based audit

3. To identify the relative strengths and weaknesses of the significant event and conventional approaches to medical audit in general practice

4. To examine the impact of each approach to medical audit on the quality of care of some marker conditions within general practice.

METHODS

Study practices

Twenty multiple-partner practices in a wide variety of localities were recruited for the study. Singlehanded practices were excluded as the method required practice

Table M1 Demographic characteristics of study practices (conventional audit arm)

Practice number	Location	Number of partners	List size	Location
1	Lincolnshire	2	3541	Village
2	Lincolnshire	3	4300	City
3	Lincolnshire	7	14000	Town
4	Lincolnshire	4	6000	Village
5	Lincolnshire	2	5471	Village
6	Manchester	6	12500	Suburban
7	Manchester	2	4000	Suburban
8	Manchester	4	7200	Suburban
9	Manchester	6	12500	Suburban
10	Manchester	4	7200	Suburban
Average		4	7671	

Table M2 Demographic characteristics of study practices (significant event arm)

Practice number	Location	Number of partners	List size	Location
1	Lincolnshire	4	5600	Village
2	Lincolnshire	4	7600	Town
3	Lincolnshire	6	11000	Town
4	Lincolnshire	3	5800	Village
5	Lincolnshire	4	5911	Village
6	Manchester	3	7300	Suburban
7	Manchester	3	7100	Suburban
8	Manchester	5	12000	Suburban
9	Manchester	3	6500	Suburban
10	Manchester	3	6000	Suburban
Average		3.8	7481	

discussion of audit results and agreement between doctors in practices to implement findings. To increase the representativeness of the practices, half were recruited from a rural area (Lincolnshire) and half were recruited from an urban area (Manchester). Within each locality an equal number of practices were randomly assigned to carry out medical audit over a one-year period using the conventional cohort-based approach or using significant event analysis. The demographic characteristics of the practices recruited in each arm of the study is given in Tables M1 and M2. In addition, information on the attitudes of participating doctors to medical audit was measured using a previously developed and validated questionnaire (Pringle et al., 1994). Practices were invited to a meeting with research workers at the end of the study to review their experience during the study year. Finally, at the conclusion of the study, all participants were asked to complete a brief questionnaire on their experience of the study and how they intended to proceed after the study.

Study requirements

Each practice in the study was asked to hold a minimum of six audit meetings over the study year, regardless of the audit method being used. They were all asked to audit the care of diabetes and doctor availability. Except for these two areas, practices made their own choices regarding what was to be audited, although they were encouraged to consider both clinical and administrative aspects of care. Audits of diabetes and doctor availability were requested from all practices to try and give us some common indicators by which to judge any changes occurring in any practice. In the event, data from the audits of doctor availability proved unusable (see page 10) but diabetes care was assessed by the research team at the start of the study, at the six-month point, and at the end of the study, for all practices. For this purpose practices were asked to grant access to their patient records and a diabetes register. A random list of 50 diabetic patients was drawn from the register and their records were examined for measures of the quality of diabetes care. Table M3 details the parameters by which diabetes care was assessed. This assessment procedure, including the random selection of patients, was repeated at the beginning, middle, and end of the study.

Conventional audit arm

Practices in the conventional audit arm of the study were asked to undertake six audits each over the course of the year. These are listed in Appendix 5. In this arm of the study, audit was conducted in the familiar pattern described in texts on medical audit. The area of audit was chosen; standards were set or adopted; performance was measured (which usually involved some special data-gathering exercise); this was compared with the standards; and a decision was reached about how to modify practice to bring performance closer to the standard(s). All audit meetings were attended by the research assistants. Although it did not prove possible for the practices to complete the audit cycle within the duration of the study, it was completed by the research team in the form of external audits of diabetes care (see page 9).

Significant event audit arm

Practices in the significant event analysis arm of the study were asked to take a radically different approach to audit based on systematic case review. Members of the practice teams were invited to meet and draw up a list of significant events for which they would all look out. They were asked to include in this list events relating to the care of diabetes and doctor availability as given on page 6 to allow comparison with the conventional audit of these areas being undertaken. All relevant team members were to be supplied with a reminder sheet of the events, the recording of which was agreed, to facilitate their recording and recall of significant events. At two-monthly intervals they would meet to discuss selected cases in a structured way. In the discussion the case would be reviewed to ascertain the quality of care given. Means of addressing any deficiencies in care were discussed and, where possible, action was agreed. Practices were supported initially with a briefing meeting to explain fully the process of significant event analysis and were also offered a list of suggested significant events (Table M4). During significant event meetings, which were

Table M3 Variables recorded for a sample of 50 patients with diabetes in each practice at the start of study, at six months and at one year, used by research assistants for the assessment of diabetes care

Diagnosis clear?
Year of diagnosis clear?
Shared care clear?
Current treatment clear?
Number of random blood sugars done in 2 years? Average number/patient?
Number of HbA1 done in 2 years? Average number/patient?
Number of fructosamines done in 2 years? Average number/patient?
Number of RBS results in 2 years? Average number/patient?
Number of HbA1 results in 2 years? Average number/patient?
Number of fructosamine results in 2 years? Average number/patient?
Average last 5 RBS? Average 5 RBS all patients?
Average last 5 HbA1? Average 5 HbA1 all patients
Average last 5 fructosamines? Average 5 fructosamines all patients?
Number of months since last blood? Average months/patient?
Number of months since last BP? Average months/patient?
Last BP systolic? Average last systolic?
Last BP diastolic? Average last diastolic?
Number of months since last weight recorded? Average months/patient?
Last weight recorded (kg)? Average last weight?
Number of months since last visual acuity? Average months last visual acuity?
Number of months since last fundoscopy recorded? Average months last fundoscopy?
Number of months since last urine albumen recorded? Average months last urine albumen?
Number of months since last foot pulses recorded? Average months last foot pulse?
Number of months since reflexes? Average months last reflexes?
Acute hypoglycaemia?
Acute hyperglycaemia?
Foot ulceration/amputation?
Stroke/TIA
Coronary or angina?
Heart failure?
Hypertension?
Hyperlipidaemia?
Claudication?
Registered blind/partial?
Retinopathy/maculopathy?
Nephropathy/urinary tract infection?
Neuropathy?

Table M4 Suggested significant events

Preventive care:
Case of whooping cough
Case of measles
Case of mumps
Unplanned pregnancy
A pregnancy with no clear recording of rubella
    immunization/immunity
Positive cervical smear
Non-accidental injury
Orchidopexy
Congenital dislocation of hip
Hearing aid (under 12)
Squint diagnosed by ophthalmologist
Diagnosis of tuberculosis
Abnormal liver function tests (alcohol)

Acute care:
Sudden unexpected death
Myocardial infarction
Cerebrovascular accident
Suicidal attempt
All new cancer diagnoses
Renal failure
Intra-uterine or perinatal death
Sudden infant death syndrome

Chronic disease:
Diabetes: registered partially sighted/blind*
           urgent visit for diabetic problem*
           diagnosis of MI, CVA or TIA*
           leg ulcer or amputation*
Asthma: urgent visit request
         hospital admission
Epilepsy: status epilepticus

Organization:
Home visit accepted but not done*
Letter received but not acted upon
Abnormal pathological result (e.g. smear) not acted upon
A breach of confidentiality
Patient changes practice without changing address
Complaint about the appointments system*
Urgent appointment request not seen in 12 hours*
Routine appointment (any doctor) not available for more
    than 2 working days*
Routine appointment for a specific doctor not available for
    more than 3 working days*
Referral letter not sent
Patient complaint reported to doctor, nurse or manager
Upset staff

* Events to be included by all study practices to test for changes and allow comparison with background audits by research assistants.
Source: This list was first published in *Audit Trends* (1994, vol. **2**, 20–24) and is reproduced with permission of the Editor.

attended by our research assistants, the practice team was encouraged to identify action as a result of the discussions and to specify how any action would be followed up.

Statistics

To enable comparisons of diabetes care at the beginning and end of the study and between the two groups of practices in the study, the Mann–Whitney U test (two-tailed z score) was used for non-parametric data and the two-tailed t-test was used for parametric data.

RESULTS

Audits of clinical care

Conventional audit practices

A. *Audits of the care of diabetes:* All 10 practices in this arm of the study succeeded in carrying out audits of their care of diabetes, although one practice was not prepared to share the findings of its audit with the research assistant. The number of parameters of diabetes care examined was very variable with some practices looking at only two parameters and others looking at 10 or more.

Five practices reviewed a sample of their diabetic patients whereas the other four (of those who shared their results) examined records of the entire population of known diabetics. Two practices confined their audit to non-insulin dependent diabetes whereas the others considered all patients with diabetes.

The most popular parameters used to audit care of diabetes were: the frequency of attendance at the practice (6/9); HbA1 (6/9); random blood sugar (6/9); weight recording (6/9); blood pressure measurement (6/9); fundoscopy (6/9); lipids/cholesterol checks (5/9); examination of feet/chiropody (4/9); urea and electrolytes (3/9); checking pulses (3/9); recording of smoking (3/9); urinary protein testing (3/9); and frequency of hospital review (3/9).

Six practices concluded from their audit that efforts needed to be made to improve the recording of the relevant parameters but in half the cases it was declared that the hospitals were mainly to blame for the relative paucity of data and decisions were made to seek improvements in the communication of results from hospital clinics. Three practices decided to design some sort of stamp for the records of patients with diabetes while three also decided to set up a diabetic mini-clinic. Two practices committed themselves to a further audit of this area of care.

B. *Audits of other clinical topics:* In addition to the 10 audits of the care of diabetes these practices conducted a total of 17 other audits of areas of clinical care (Appendix 5). Of these the majority (13) were audits of chronic disease management including: hypertension (3), asthma (2), hormone replacement therapy (HRT) (2), patients on vitamin B_{12} (2), patients on lithium (2), thyroid disease (1), and use of topical steroids long term (1). Another audit concerned long-term benzodiazepine

prescribing but was not related to any specific disease or group of diseases. Two audits (one of oral contraceptive practice and one of cervical cytology screening) were related to disease prevention, though the three on hypertension and the two on HRT could also be construed as being concerned with disease prevention. One audit was of an acute illness, namely urinary tract infection in women of child-bearing age.

As a result of these audits, a wide variety of changes were suggested. The duration and nature of the study did not allow us to ascertain whether or not such changes actually did occur, though the results of the exit questionnaire at least are encouraging (see page 13). Most of the clinical audits led to resolutions to improve follow-up, in most instances by closer monitoring of laboratory parameters of the disease or its treatment. Ten of the audits led to the introduction of some new protocol or practice procedure. In two of them this involved the setting up of a call/recall procedure. Five of the audits led to a decision to strive to improve record keeping including the need for better recording of the initial diagnosis. One audit (of asthma) led to a decision to improve patient education. In the case of another (of thyroid diseases) it was decided that further discussion was needed. One of the audits of lithium led to a decision to seek clarification from the hospital regarding responsibilities of the practice and the hospital in patient monitoring. While in most instances audits led to resolution to do more and better, in one instance (that of the audit of urinary tract infection) it was decided to do less, namely to abandon the pre-treatment midstream urine specimens in most instances.

Significant event practices

A. *Significant events in the care of diabetes:* Forty-nine significant events in the care of patients with diabetes were noted but of these only 16 were chosen for discussion at the significant events meeting. Four of those discussed related to the initial diagnosis and in none of these was any scope for earlier diagnosis identified. Ten related to complications of diabetes including four about patients who had to have amputations; two concerned patients with ocular complications of diabetes; one concerned a sixth nerve palsy; one concerned a co-existing infection; one concerned an episode of ketoacidosis; and another concerned an episode of hypoglycaemia. The remaining four related to episodes of poor diabetic control. By and large these significant events did not reveal major flaws in the practices' procedures for the care of diabetes, although there were several in which the patient's failure to comply with requests for follow-up appointments was felt to be the main factor in the genesis of the significant event. In one instance, blindness resulted from diabetes, in spite of an ophthalmic referral prior to the onset of blindness. This was felt to be due to considerable delays on the hospital side in booking outpatient appointments and a failure to prioritize among those patients referred.

B. *Other significant events in the care of patients:* A further 489 events pertaining to clinical care in areas other than diabetes were noted. Of these, 161 were discussed at significant event meetings (Appendix 2). Of these, 41 concerned sudden death or cardiovascular or cerebrovascular disease; 31 concerned events in the care of patients with cancer (many around the diagnosis); 35 concerned a variety of chronic diseases including the 16 events relating to diabetes and its care; 15 related to contraception and other events in the arena of women's health; 12 related to suicide, attempted suicide, violent deaths and other physical trauma; 13 related to various infections including 4 around cases of meningitis; and 4 seemed to arise primarily from problems at the primary–secondary care interface. Beyond these broad categories there were isolated events pertaining to virtually every area of clinical care imaginable.

For 80 of the significant events discussed, either a decision was reached that no action was required to address the problems discussed, or no decision on any action was made. In 35 instances a decision was made, however, to institute a new procedure or protocol in the practice to deal with the deficiencies exposed. In the case of a further 13, rather than institute a whole new policy there was a decision to issue a new instruction to practice staff (in four cases this meant administrative staff and in nine this meant doctors). In 34 instances a less firm decision was reached and discussions concluded with general exhortations (of varying levels of specificity) to staff to try harder to do better. In 11 instances the decision was to hold further meetings or discussions; in 9 instances it was decided to seek more information; and in 5 it was decided to monitor the situation or give the matter further consideration. In another 9 cases it was decided to contact the hospital concerned usually because it was felt that only the hospital could have improved the care given and in three instances it was decided to contact other bodies such as the family health services authority. In 4 cases a decision to inform patients or to improve patient education was the outcome and in 1 case it was decided that staff education was required. In 4 cases it was decided to conduct a conventional audit.

Comparison of conventional audit and significant event audit practices

As was to be expected, conventional audit practices covered fewer areas of clinical practice than did significant event analysis practices but those covered were done so in much greater depth. It is notable, though, that the range of areas covered was even narrower than it could have been and certain aspects of prevention and chronic diseases care predominated. Furthermore, although most conventional audits led to more than one decision being made, the range of types of decision made was also rather confined. In over half, the decisions did involve the introduction of new procedures or protocols but only rarely was it decided to involve others in the solution of problems identified (the range of which was also rather restricted).

In contrast, significant event practices covered a much wider range of clinical areas extending into terminal care, acute diseases, women's health and most clinical disciplines. Furthermore, they covered a wide range of relatively rare but very important events such as cancer diagnoses, sudden deaths and violent deaths. This method of auditing also allowed the review of the care of difficult or awkward patients *per se*. The range of deficiencies in care exposed was also very wide and often extended beyond the immediate primary carers. Hence deficiencies in secondary care were, perhaps, more often

the subject of discussion. Similarly, the range of changes suggested or solutions offered was correspondingly wide, although there often appeared a readiness to accept the status quo or to defer action. There was also less specificity about the solutions suggested. Where definitive action was proposed this was, in many instances, limited in scope. Quite often the decision was reached that nothing more could be done. As significant event discussions are not confined to matters within the control of the practice, the action proposed not infrequently entailed involving others in any planned improvements in the quality of care.

Audits of practice administration

Conventional audit practices

A. Audits of doctor availability: At the outset all practices were asked to carry out an audit of doctor availability. Conventional audit practices were asked to conduct a formal audit of appointment procedures, while significant event practices were asked to look out for significant events relating to doctor availability. All 10 conventional audit practices conducted some form of audit on the question of doctor availability. Six of these audits took the form of seeking patients' views (and in two instances also staff views) on the operation of the appointment system. Two of the other practices carried out retrospective examinations of workload data on the numbers of patients seen during the previous year. The other two practices also looked at work flow patterns, particularly in relation to any mismatch between number of appointments offered and number of patients seen, though they did so prospectively. Generally results seemed to indicate acceptable performance against the practices' own (generally fairly stringent) standards and a high level of patient satisfaction. Only two practices felt the need to change their procedures immediately on the findings of their audit. Several others did agree to seek further information and/or to re-audit but no commitment to any particular change in their procedures was agreed during the study. Generally speaking the decisions were to leave matters well alone regarding the appointments system. Some of these practices actually did dual audits in this area. Thus one practice looked at availability of appointments and at patients' telephone access to the practice. Others used combinations of direct observations of actual performance and views of patients and/or staff as expressed in satisfaction surveys.

B. Other administrative audits: In addition to the required audits of doctor availability 20 other administrative type audits were carried out by conventional audit practices (Appendices 5 and 6). One of these, although ostensibly about patient satisfaction, was also primarily about satisfaction with the appointment system. Two further audits were of treatment room activity and concerned primarily nurse availability and another was overtly concerned with nurse appointments. In yet another practice they conducted an audit of individual doctors' workloads in addition to their audit of the appointment system. Of the remaining 16 audits, 11 were in areas relating to health promotion and disease prevention but when conducted from the administrative point of view these tended to concentrate on the meeting of immunization targets (2 audits), ensuring all fees were earned and paid (4 audits), or ensuring compliance with the new contract (3 audits). Two of the other audits related to referrals (one to outpatients; one to x-ray). Two others related to prescribing matters (one to patients' prescription requests and another to a practice formulary). The last remaining audit was really a full staffing review.

Broadly speaking, practices were pleased with the results of these audits and in 4 cases no change flowed from the audit. In 4 audits the sole decision was to review again and in 2 cases the results suggested such success in meeting the original standard set that the outcome was a decision to set a new, higher standard. In 6 cases there was a decision to institute a new procedure or protocol and in one case a decision to set up a whole new clinic. In two further cases the decision was just generally to improve, although in another two the exhortation was specifically to improve recording. Three audits led to staff changes, including in two instances employing new staff, and in one other the decision was made to increase staff training. In one case the decision reached was to contact the hospital.

Significant event practices

A. Audits of doctor availability: Among significant event practices, 51 events concerning doctor availability were noted, of which 15 were discussed. Of these, 5 concerned the appointment system specifically. One concerning nurse availability also arose and there was one concerning a failure to visit. In the cases of non-availability of surgery consultations two incidents arose from doctors being called out on emergencies and none resulted in a patient complaint. One of the commoner ways in which such lack of availability came to attention was by virtue of the fact that patients had to stand owing to lack of seating in the waiting area.

B. Other administrative audits: Significant event practices noted a total of 345 administrative events other than those concerning doctor availability of which 94 were discussed at significant event meetings (Appendix 2). Sixteen were deemed to be errors of omission (i.e. something not done that should have been) and 5 were deemed to be errors of commission (i.e. things done that should not have been). Only 5 concerned the appointments system and none of these resulted in a patient complaint. There were, however, 17 events discussed that concerned a patient having complained, although there were also 4 events discussed where it was decided that it was the patients' (unreasonable) behaviour that was to blame. Eleven other events discussed arose in connection with the prescribing or dispensing of drugs. Beyond these the range was very wide with matters covered including practice policies or procedures (6 events discussed); home visits, emergencies and out-of-hours calls (3 events discussed); premises (3 events discussed); rotas (4 events discussed); meetings (2 events discussed); confidentiality (3 events discussed); records (5 events discussed); secondary care (6 events discussed); and a whole variety of other even less commonly discussed matters.

Interestingly, 15 personnel matters were listed but none was ever discussed.

Following discussion of these administrative significant event audits, no decision was made in the case of 15 and a decision that no action was required was made in respect of a further 5. In 5 cases it was decided to seek further information or ideas and in 12 more the decision was deferred for further discussion or a working party was to be set up. In 19 cases the main decision was to tighten up existing practice systems or procedures, whereas for a further 30 the decision was to institute new policies or procedures. In 17 cases the decision was to educate, inform or instruct the patient. In 16 cases new instructions were issued to doctors, nurses, and other members of the primary care team. In 13 instances the decision was to contact some other person (such as the health visitor) the family health services authority or the hospital. In 8 cases the result was a decision to improve records or communication more generally. In two cases additional staff training was suggested and in one other a decision was made to appoint a new member of staff (a new nurse). Finally, in two instances the decisions included one to conduct a further audit later.

Comparison of conventional audit and significant event audit practices

As with the clinical audits, significant event analysis of administrative events covered a much wider range of problems, though perhaps in less depth, than did the conventional audits. Also, as before, the range of actions flowing from conventional audits was rather more limited in scope than those flowing from significant event analyses, although in this case there was no obvious change suggested by either type of audit in many instances.

Background audits to measure changes in quality of care

In addition to the audits conducted by the practices themselves, the research assistants also conducted audits of the care of diabetes mellitus and of doctor availability at the start of the study, after six months, and at the end of the study. These two areas were to be used as markers of change occurring as a result of audit going on in the practices.

Care of diabetes mellitus

When it came to assessing the care of diabetes six key variables of the list of parameters measured at the beginning, middle, and end of the study (see Methods) were identified as discriminant markers of quality of care. These were:

- number of random blood sugars (RBS) in the medical records over the past 2 years

- number of glycosylated haemoglobin or fructosamine results in the medical records over the past 2 years

- the mean level of the last five random blood sugars

- the mean level of the last five glycosylated haemoglobin results

Table R1 Changes in six key parameters of diabetes care over the course of the study (n = number of patients with any valid reading for the parameter)

	Start of study year (n)	End of study year (n)
Mean number of RBS results recorded in the medical records over the past two years	3.27 (808)	3.43 (836)
Mean number of HbA1 results recorded in the medical records over the past two years	2.40 (562)	2.24 (628)
Mean of the mean of the past five RBS results recorded in the medical records	11.80 (616)	11.43 (699)
Mean of the mean of the past five HbA1 results recorded in the medical records	9.97 (394)	9.03 (418)
Mean of the last systolic blood pressure recorded in the medical records	148.16 (900)	148.42 (931)
Mean of the last diastolic blood pressure recorded in the medical records	82.46 (898)	82.02 (929)

- the last recorded systolic blood pressure
- the last recorded diastolic blood pressure.

It was found that for each of these variables the number of medical records with a valid reading increased over the year of the study (Table R1). By the end of the year 93% of records of diabetic patients had a blood pressure reading in their notes, although only 41% had had, by then, five HbA1 results. For five of the key parameters of performance the practices improved over the year of the study. More RBS readings had been made and RBS and HbA1 readings were on average lower at the study end, although this improvement was statistically significant only in the case of HbA1 readings (two-tailed t-test; t = 5.64; p<0.0001). Diastolic blood pressure readings were also marginally lower at the end of the study. Mean systolic blood pressure rose by 0.26 mmHg but this difference was not statistically significant. Likewise the number of HbA1 readings fell in the past two years from 2.40 to 2.24, but this difference was also not statistically significant

Comparison of conventional audit and significant event analysis practices

Table R2 shows how the conventional audit and significant event practices compared in terms of the key

parameters of diabetes care over the course of the study. No significant difference was demonstrated between the two groups of practices in terms of the recording of variables. However, in terms of performance some significant differences were noted. Practices in the conventional audit arm of the study were found at the beginning of the study to have had significantly fewer RBS readings within the past two years (Mann–Whitney U test; two-tailed; z = −6.96; p<0.0001); fewer HbA1 readings (Mann–Whitney U test; two-tailed; z = −5.07; p<0.0001); and higher levels of RBS recorded (two-tailed t-test; t = 2.01; p = 0.04). The mean level of HbA1 found in conventional audit practices was not significantly higher than it was in the significant event practices.

These differences persisted and similarly significant differences were found between the two groups of patients at the end of the study period. Thus there were fewer RBS results (Mann–Whitney U test; two-tailed; z = −2.98; p = 0.003); fewer HbA1 results (Mann–Whitney U test; two-tailed; z = −4.20; p<0.0001); and higher levels of RBS (two-tailed t-test; t = 2.15; p = 0.03) in the conventional audit practices.

Practices in the conventional audit arm of the study improved their level of recording of RBS and HbA1 over the year. Significant event practices slightly reduced theirs. None of these differences, though, was statistically significant.

Patients in both groups showed a tightening in mean glycaemic control with no significant difference between the two groups. Patients in the significant event practices showed a small but insignificant rise in systolic blood pressure (difference of mean = 0.67; n.s.) but otherwise mean blood pressure dropped slightly with no significant difference between the two groups demonstrated.

Doctor availability

It was originally intended that a comparable background audit of doctors' availability would be conducted. In the event, the variability of practice arrangements for determining and allocating consulting times with doctors was such that our proposed standardized audits could not be completed in a way that gave fairly comparable measures of doctor availability. We were unable to establish a common platform on which to compare the performance of all practices and so the attempt was abandoned.

Attitudes to audit

Table R3 shows that overall the study doctors had very positive attitudes to medical audit. Four out of five see it as an effective means of improving the quality of medical care and three-quarters think it reveals interesting things about their practices. Twenty-six (45%) strongly or moderately agreed that systematic review of single cases could tell you a lot about your practice in general while a similar number were non-committal on this point. Those practices in the significant events arm of the study were better disposed, on average, to the idea of single case review (Table R4). Study practices had, overall, more positive attitudes to medical audit than did a much larger sample of unselected practices

Table R2 Changes in the six key parameters of diabetes care in the two arms of the study (n = number of patients with any valid reading for the parameter—maximum 500)

	Start of study year		End of study year	
	Conventional audit arm (n)	Significant event arm (n)	Conventional audit arm (n)	Significant event arm (n)
Mean number of RBS results recorded in the medical records over the past two years	2.81 (400)	3.72 (408)	3.20 (398)	3.64 (438)
Mean number of HbA1 results recorded in the medical records over the past two years	2.07 (288)	2.75 (274)	2.02 (329)	2.47 (299)
Mean of the mean of the past five RBS results recorded in the medical records	12.17 (291)	11.48 (325)	11.80 (328)	11.11 (371)
Mean of the mean of the past five HbA1 results recorded in the medical records	10.14 (194)	9.80 (200)	8.99 (211)	9.06 (207)
Mean of the last systolic blood pressure recorded	148.64 (444)	147.69 (456)	148.48 (458)	148.36 (473)
Mean of the last diastolic blood pressure recorded	82.63 (443)	82.30 (455)	81.94 (457)	82.11 (472)

surveyed previously (Pringle et al., 1994). This difference appears to be largely due to a much more positive attitude to medical audit among the practices in the significant event arm of the study. Similarly, rural doctors in the study appeared to have more positive attitudes to audit overall (Table R5), a finding confirmed by the previous larger survey of unselected practices in urban and rural localities (Pringle et al., 1994).

Success in meeting the study requirements

Doing this study has afforded our researchers the opportunity to observe at close range 20 practices conducting medical audit over a one-year period using two different models of medical audit. As well as being able to describe the audits carried out and the conclusions reached from these, and being able to attempt some measure of outcomes for quality of care in limited spheres, this study has also given us some insights into how the practices function more globally. We have, in particular, been able to observe their success or otherwise in struggling to meet the considerable demands of carrying on medical audit. These observations have been supplemented by comments from participants made at meetings held at the conclusion of the study (exit meetings) and on the basis of a questionnaire completed by participants at the close of the study (the exit questionnaire). It has also proven possible on the basis of these observations and comments to make some informed judgements regarding those factors likely to be associated with greater success in carrying on with medical audit.

In this regard, we can discern two sorts of measure of success. There are the more task-focused measures which are simply to do with whether or not participants were able to comply with the requirements we placed on them when they were recruited to the study. Thus, we could

look at how many audits were done; how many meetings were held by the practice; how many people attended the meetings; and how much change in the practice appeared to be evoked by the audit process. The second sort of measure of success requires more qualitative judgements by the participants and the researchers regarding the quality of audits conducted; the less tangible benefits to the practice of auditing (such as team building); and whether or not real change did occur. We also looked at the success of the primary health care teams in terms of good team working and improved communication, as these benefits appeared to accrue even when, by the more limited task-oriented measures, the practices appeared not to be performing so well.

Conventional audit arm

In both Manchester and Lincolnshire audit meetings were generally carried out as part of regular practice meetings (8/10) and attendance was generally good (Table R6). Only one of the practices assigned by randomization to this arm of the study expressed a preference for the other method of medical audit (significant event analysis). Eight of the practices in this arm were computerized.

Six of the practices held meetings at the required intervals (minimum two monthly). All practices involved all doctors and in 8 out of 10 the practice manager was involved—in one practice the practice manager took the chair. In general, though, the lead in audit was taken by one or more of the partners—sometimes in a fairly loose and flexible rotation. In those practices where only one doctor seemed to take the lead, more organizational difficulties arose. Staff other than doctors were involved in 6 out of 10 practices. These non-medical staff all expressed some reservations or concerns about what was involved in audit, although these seemed to diminish over time.

Table R3 Responses of study doctors to paired statements on attitudes to medical audit (%=percentage of valid responses)

Topic	Statement	Strongly or moderately agree n (%)	Slightly agree or disagree n (%)	Moderately or strongly disagree n (%)
Quality of care	Medical audit is an effective means of improving the quality of medical care	48 (79)	12 (20)	1 (2)
	Medical audit is not necessary to ensure the quality of care	8 (13)	23 (38)	30 (49)
Time	Time spent on medical audit is time well spent	31 (51)	28 (46)	2 (3)
	Medical audit is a waste of time	2 (3)	12 (20)	47 (77)
Interest	Medical audit reveals interesting things about your practice	46 (75)	13 (21)	2 (3)
	Medical audit is boring	9 (15)	27 (44)	25 (41)
Leadership	Medical audit is a professionally led attempt to ensure the quality of care	41 (67)	18 (30)	2 (3)
	Medical audit is another bureaucratic ploy to limit the clinical freedom of doctors	3 (5)	25 (41)	33 (54)
Sample size	In order to get a true picture you need to audit a large sample of cases	12 (20)	23 (38)	26 (43)
	The size of the sample is not crucial to what can be learnt from an audit	28 (46)	18 (30)	15 (25)
Case review	Systematic review of single cases can tell you a lot about your practice in general	26 (45)	26 (45)	6 (10)
	Just reviewing single cases is too woolly and vague to be considered as proper audit	14 (23)	27 (44)	20 (33)

Four practices experienced some difficulty in completing audits, although 9 out of 10 did complete the requisite six audits by the end of the study—one practice having conducted a long and complex audit over four months that we counted as two audits. The remaining practice completed only four audits owing to an unexpected and major disruption to the life of the practice.

Significant event arm

In this group of practices, too, significant event audit was, in most instances (8/10), carried out as part of regular practice meetings (Table R7). Practices in this arm of the study generally experienced more difficulties with meeting the study requirements. In only three practices did all the general practitioners attend all the audit meetings. Two practices encountered major difficulties and managed to hold only three of the required six meetings. Many of these difficulties were logistic (for example, relating to illness of doctors, extensive other commitments) but some, it must be conceded, might relate to the challenges of the method, as in five practices some information concerning significant events was withheld from the researchers because it was deemed "too sensitive".

Six of the practices (3 in Manchester; 3 in Lincolnshire) held meetings at the required intervals (minimum two-monthly). Practice managers attended meetings in 7 out of 10 practices and, where present, were seen to take a full and active part in proceedings; that is, they were not just functioning as an administrative/secretarial observer. As in the conventional arm, partners tended to take the lead role, although in one practice it was the practice manager who chaired all the meetings. Leadership in this arm of the study was often more fluid and of a generally participative nature. Staff other than doctors were involved in 5 out of 10 practices with nurses being in attendance in all 5 of these and clerical staff being involved in 2 out of the 10 practices. The involvement of additional staff was observed to give a broader perspective to the audit and resulted in a wider range of issues being considered. Some team members did express concern about this form of audit. Some nurses were concerned about the safeguards for confidentiality and were hesitant about the presence of "outsiders" (specifically the research assistants). Some reception staff not involved in the process were concerned that the method would encourage a "witch hunt" to find someone to blame when things had been seen to go wrong.

Table R4 Mean scores in response to paired attitudinal statements concerning medical audit (strongly agree = 1; strongly disagree = 6) of study doctors

Topic	Statement	Conventional arm (n = 28)	Significant arm (n = 34)	All study doctors (n = 62)
Quality of care	Medical audit is an effective means of improving the quality of medical care	2.36	1.67	1.98
	Medical audit is not necessary to ensure the quality of care	3.75	4.39	4.10
Time	Time spent on medical audit is time well spent	2.89	2.30	2.57
	Medical audit is a waste of time	4.71	5.27	5.02
Interest	Medical audit reveals interesting things about your practice	2.32	1.76	2.02
	Medical audit is boring	3.61	4.27	3.97
Leadership	Medical audit is a professionally led attempt to ensure the quality of care	2.57	1.91	2.21
	Medical audit is another bureaucratic ploy to limit the clinical freedom of doctors	4.07	4.85	4.49
Sample size	In order to get a true picture you need to audit a large sample of cases	3.64	4.18	3.93
	The size of the sample is not crucial to what can be learnt from an audit	3.36	2.97	3.05
Case review	Systematic review of single cases can tell you a lot about your practice in general	3.18	2.47	2.81
	Just reviewing single cases is too woolly and vague to be considered as proper audit	3.39	3.91	3.67

Exit questionnaire

Perceived benefits from the audit process

The responses to the exit questionnaire were generally positive about the benefits of audit with a large proportion of participants claiming to have benefited from taking part in audit within a structured and facilitated framework. Eighty-nine per cent of respondents to the exit questionnaire thought they would definitely or probably continue with regular audit (Table R8); 86% reported that decisions reached had been implemented at least "some of the time" and no doctor reported that no decisions had been implemented; 63% believed their personal audit skills had definitely or probably increased and 25% were entirely sure that necessary change had occurred over the period of the study; 68% felt that patient care had definitely or probably improved. Taking part also had positive effects on the working of the primary health care team with over 70% of the general practitioners responding agreeing that communication within, and efficiency or organization of the practice had definitely or probably improved during the study period. There were no significant differences in the responses of doctors in either conventional or significant event arms of the study or from those practising in the rural or urban settings (Table R9).

Features of the process associated with successful audit

The second part of the exit questionnaire explored the participants' views on the features of the audit process that might be associated with greater or lesser effectiveness. The results of this part of the questionnaire are shown in Table R8. Over 90% agreed, to some extent, that successful audit required a practice leader on audit (not necessarily a doctor); a supportive practice team; an enthusiastic practice manager; trust within the team; re-audit at intervals; explicit agreed standards; protocol development; feedback; and appropriate resources (specifically time, money and staff). The need to implement change as a consequence of the audit process was stated to be very or moderately important by over 90% of respondents. Extensive audit experience and external facilitation were not seen as quite so vital to the success of audit. In relation to these judgements there were also no significant differences between arms of the study or locations of the practices.

Exit meetings

The exit questionnaire was designed to capture the impressions from both arms of the study and, consequently, sought responses to general statements about audit. This

Table R5 Mean scores in response to paired attitudinal statements concerning medical audit (strongly agree = 1; strongly disagree = 6) of urban and rural doctors in the study

Topic	Statement	Lincolnshire (n = 32)	Manchester (n = 30)	All study doctors (n = 62)
Quality of care	Medical audit is an effective means of improving the quality of medical care	1.91	2.07	1.98
	Medical audit is not necessary to ensure the quality of care	4.31	3.86	4.10
Time	Time spent on medical audit is time well spent	2.50	2.66	2.57
	Medical audit is a waste of time	5.22	4.76	5.02
Interest	Medical audit reveals interesting things about your practice	1.81	2.24	2.02
	Medical audit is boring	4.00	3.93	3.97
Leadership	Medical audit is a professionally led attempt to ensure the quality of care	2.25	2.17	2.21
	Medical audit is another bureaucratic ploy to limit the clinical freedom of doctors	4.56	4.41	4.49
Sample size	In order to get a true picture you need to audit a large sample of cases	3.84	4.03	3.93
	The size of the sample is not crucial to what can be learnt from an audit	3.19	2.90	3.05
Case review	Systematic review of single cases can tell you a lot about your practice in general	2.90	2.71	2.81
	Just reviewing single cases is too woolly and vague to be considered as proper audit	3.75	3.59	3.67

may be why it failed to show any significant differences between different doctor cohorts. The exit meetings were more flexibly run and picked up rather more on the contrasts between the two different approaches to medical audit.

Conventional audit arm

Most members of the practice teams in this arm of the study expressed satisfaction with the process of audit and with the areas selected for audit. Little difficulty was experienced in choosing audit topics, although audits were generally done on areas considered by conventional wisdom to be 'problem areas'. Practices did not appear to have a process for generating their own list(s) of problem areas. Conventional audit was generally seen to be a straightforward affair by participating practices, although clerical staff required to carry out data collection without any other involvement in the audit process felt audit to be a chore. Such difficulties as did occur appeared more related to external factors (such as communication difficulties) rather than factors intrinsic to this method of medical audit. Such logistic obstacles were thoroughly discussed at audit meetings. The word audit was unpopular at the start of the study and remained so at the end, but by then the underlying concept was perceived as less threatening.

Seven out of 10 practices in this arm considered audit to have acted as a catalyst for favourable change with change occurring most frequently in key areas such as protocol development. The audit of diabetes care was singled out as the area where the greatest number of favourable changes had been made. Decisions made at audit meetings were implemented in 8 out of 10 practices. All practices in this arm of the study expressed a desire to continue audit after the end of the study. Most felt a level of three to four audits per year would be an appropriate number to aim for.

Significant event arm

More difficulties were expressed in relation to significant event audit, although the difficulties did lessen with familiarity with the method. More guidance in choosing audit topics was advocated and some teams would have valued more guidance in defining a significant event. Many expressed the wish that they could have spent more time discussing events (though significant event meetings generally lasted 60 to 90 minutes). Participants generally liked the formality of the significant event discussions and found it preferable to the more traditional practice of having informal discussions in corridors or over coffee. That said, it was also apparent that some events could not be held

Table R6 Attendances at meetings held at two-monthly intervals (conventional audit practices)

Practices	Partners	Nurses	Manager	Others
Practice 1	2 (2)	1	–	Trainee
	2 (2)	1	1	–
	2 (2)	2	1	–
	2 (2)	–	–	–
	2 (2)	–	1	–
	2 (2)	–	1	–
Practice 2	2 (3)	–	1	–
	3 (3)	1	1	–
	3 (3)	1	1	–
	3 (3)	1	1	–
	3 (3)	1	1	–
	3 (3)	1	1	–
Practice 3	5 (7)	–	1	Trainee
	5 (7)	3	1	–
	6 (7)	1	1	–
	6 (7)	–	1	Locum
	6 (7)	–	1	–
Practice 4	3 (4)	–	1	
	3 (4)	–	1	–
	3 (4)	–	1	–
	4 (4)	–	1	–
	3 (4)	–	1	–
Practice 5	2 (2)	1	–	–
	2 (2)	1	–	–
	2 (2)	1	–	–
	2 (2)	–	–	1 Receptionist
	2 (2)	–	–	2 Receptionists/ 1 Health visitor
	2 (2)	1	–	–
Practice 6	1 (6)	–	–	1 Secretary
	5 (6)	2	1	–
	5 (6)	2	1	–
	5 (6)	–	1	–
	6 (6)	–	1	–
	6 (6)	–	1	–
Practice 7	3 (3)	–	1	–
	2 (3)	–	–	–
	2 (2)	–	–	–
	2 (2)	–	–	–
	1 (2)	–	–	–
	2 (2)	–	–	–
(*Note:* One partner retired)				
Practice 8	4 (4)	–	1	Trainee
	3 (4)	–	1	Trainee
	2 (3)	–	1	Trainee
No further meetings— Partner died				
Practice 9	2 (5)	–	–	–
	6 (6)	–	–	–
	5 (5)	–	–	–
(*Note:* One partner retired)				
7 audits performed and discussed at three meetings				
Practice 10	3 (4)	–	0	Trainee
	3 (4)	–	0	Trainee
	3 (4)	–	0	Trainee
	3 (4)	–	0	Trainee
	4 (4)	–	0	Trainee
	4 (4)	–	0	Trainee

over until the formal meeting. Sometimes team members had discussed events while they were 'hot' and had already implemented changes rendering discussion at a formal meeting less necessary. The complete openness and trust about potentially sensitive matters and matters of deep professional pride required for this method to work proved difficult for some teams, particularly initially.

Overall, though, 9 out of the 10 practices expressed satisfaction with the process and considered this form of audit both beneficial and educational. Most expressed the belief that communication, confidence and trust within the team had improved over the life of the study. However, team members excluded from the process (most often clerical/reception staff) tended to feel more threatened by it. Nurses and other ancillary staff who had attended significant event meetings expressed the view that this had helped to improve their general understanding of patients and clinical management decisions. Some members of practice teams said that significant event auditing was more motivating than conventional auditing. Most practices (9/10) expressed a desire to continue to audit after the end of the study, although many anticipated difficulties over finding time for audit meetings.

Role of the practice manager

Conventional audit arm

The practice manager attended meetings in 8 out of 10 practices. It was noted that where practice managers attended they had a central role in organizing the meeting. All practice managers were observed to be strongly committed to audit and several had had previous experience of audit/quality assurance from either industry or the health service. Practice managers tended to be very task/goal orientated and were committed to achieving results and seeing to it that decisions were implemented. In 9 out of the 10 practices the practice manager was solely responsible for audits of purely administrative matters and in the other the practice manager worked jointly with a general practitioner on these audits.

Significant event arm

One practice in the significant event arm of the study did not have a practice manager, although much of the role was assumed by the senior receptionist. However, she did not attend audit meetings. In 7 out of the 9 remaining practices the practice manager attended all audit meetings and was observed to take a full and active part. Indeed, in one practice the practice manager chaired all the audit meetings. In one practice the practice manager only attended when administrative significant events had come up and in the other the practice manager never attended. In this last practice no administrative events ever came up for discussion.

Table R7 Attendances at meetings held at two-monthly intervals (significant event practices)

Practices	Partners	Nurses	Manager	Others
Practice 1	2 (3)	2	1	–
	1 (3)	2	1	–
	2 (3)	2	1	–
	3 (3)	4	1	–
	2 (3)	2	1	–
	2 (3)	4	–	–
Practice 2	4 (4)	3	1	–
	3 (4)	3	1	–
	4 (4)	3	1	–
	4 (4)	2	1	Trainee
	4 (4)	2	1	Trainee
	4 (4)	1	1	Trainee
Practice 3	3 (6)	1	1	Visiting GP
				Trainee, secretary, receptionist
	5 (6)	2	1	Secretary, receptionist
	4 (5)	2	1	Trainee, secretary, receptionist
	3 (5)	1	1	Student, secretary, receptionist
	4 (6)	3	1	Trainee, secretary, receptionist
	6 (6)	–	–	Secretary/receptionist
Practice 4	4 (4)	–	1	–
	4 (4)	–	1	–
	4 (4)	–	1	–
	3 (4)	–	–	–
	4 (4)	–	1	–
	4 (4)	–	1	–
Practice 5	4 (4)	1	1	Trainee
	4 (4)	1	1	Trainee
	4 (4)	2	1	Trainee, student
	4 (4)	2	–	Trainee, visiting GP
	4 (4)	1	1	Trainee
	4 (4)	2	1	Trainee
Practice 6	3 (3)	–	1	–
	2 (3)	–	1	–
	3 (3)	–	1	–
	3 (3)	–	1	–
	3 (3)	–	1	–
	3 (3)	–	1	–
Practice 7	3 (3)	–	–	–
	3 (3)	–	–	–
	2 (2)	–	–	–
	3 (3)	–	–	–
	3 (3)	–	–	–
	3 (3)	–	–	–
Practice 8	5 (5)	–	1	–
	5 (5)	–	1	–
	4 (5)	–	1	–
	4 (5)	–	–	–
	3 (5)	–	–	–
	3 (5)	–	–	–
Practice 9	4 (4)	2	1	Secretary/trainee
	4 (4)	2	1	Secretary/trainee
	4 (4)	2	1	Secretary/trainee
Practice 10	3 (3)	–	–	–
	3 (3)	–	–	–
	3 (3)	–	–	–

Practices 9 and 10 had only 3 meetings, owing to cancellations.

Table R8 Responses to exit questionnaire (n = 59)

(a) *Benefits of audit*

	Definitely n (%)	Probably n (%)	Unsure n (%)	No n (%)
Do you think that taking part in the study has increased communication in the primary health care team (PHCT)?	16 (27)	30 (51)	8 (14)	5 (9)
Has it increased the PHCT's confidence in auditing?	13 (22)	36 (61)	7 (12)	3 (5)
Has it provoked necessary change?	15 (25)	28 (48)	11 (19)	5 (9)
Has it improved patient care?	8 (14)	32 (54)	17 (29)	2 (3)
Has it improved the efficiency of organization of the practice?	8 (14)	34 (58)	12 (20)	5 (9)
Do you think your personal level of audit skills has increased	18 (31)	19 (32)	14 (24)	8 (14)
Do you intend to continue regular auditing?	31 (53)	21 (36)	7 (12)	0

(b) *Implementation*

	All of the time	Most of the time	Some of the time	A few times	Hardly ever	Never
Have decisions made at audit meetings been successfully implemented?	2 (3)	25 (43)	23 (40)	7 (12)	1 (2)	0

(c) *Features required for success*

Which of these features are required to facilitate successful audit in primary care?	Very important	Moderately important	Unsure	Not important
Practice audit leader	28 (48)	28 (48)	2 (3)	1 (2)
Supportive practice team	35 (59)	22 (37)	2 (3)	0
Trust/openness in PHCT	33 (56)	23 (39)	3 (5)	0
Re-auditing after change	35 (59)	23 (39)	3 (5)	0
Feedback of results to PHCT	43 (73)	16 (27)	0	0
Sufficient resources (time, money, staff)	47 (80)	11 (19)	2 (3)	0
Extensive audit experience	4 (7)	26 (44)	13 (22)	16 (27)
Enthusiastic practice manager	24 (41)	27 (46)	6 (10)	2 (3)
Previously agreed standards against which performance can be measured	22 (37)	30 (51)	5 (9)	2 (3)
Protocols	25 (42)	25 (42)	7 (12)	2 (3)
Implementing necessary change as a result of audit	35 (58)	21 (36)	3 (5)	0
The presence of an external facilitator	5 (9)	17 (29)	27 (46)	10 (17)

Table R9 Mean responses to exit questionnaire by study doctors by study arm and location

	Conventional audit (n=28)	Significant event audit (n=31)	Lincolnshire (n=32)	Manchester (n=27)	All (n=59)
Questions with the scale 1–4 (definitely=1, no=4)					
Do you think that taking part in the study has increased communication in the primary health care team?	2.07	2.00	1.84	2.26	2.03
Has it increased the PHCT's confidence in auditing?	1.89	2.10	2.00	2.00	2.00
Has it provoked necessary change?	2.21	2.00	2.16	2.04	2.10
Has it improved patient care?	2.39	2.06	2.13	2.33	2.22
Has it improved the efficiency or organization of the practice?	2.21	2.26	2.31	2.15	2.24
Do you think your personal level of audit skills has increased?	1.96	2.42	2.25	2.15	2.20
Do you intend to continue regular auditing?	1.57	1.61	1.44	1.78	1.59
Question with scale 1–6 (all of the time=1; never=6)					
Have decisions made at audit meetings been successfully implemented?	2.63	2.68	2.63	2.69	2.66
Questions with scale 1–4 (very important=1; not important=1)					
Which of the following features are required to facilitate audit in primary care?					
Practice audit leader	1.64	1.55	1.59	1.59	1.59
Supportive practice team	1.54	1.35	1.34	1.56	1.44
Trust/openness in PHCT	1.68	1.32	1.41	1.59	1.49
Re-auditing after change	1.50	1.35	1.38	1.48	1.42
Feedback of results to PHCT	1.32	1.23	1.19	1.37	1.27
Sufficient resources (time, money, staff)	1.25	1.19	1.16	1.30	1.22
Extensive audit experience	2.89	2.52	2.63	2.78	2.69
Enthusiastic practice manager	1.75	1.77	1.69	1.85	1.76
Previously agreed standards against which performance can be measured	1.64	1.90	1.72	1.84	1.78
Protocols	1.68	1.84	1.78	1.74	1.76
Implementing necessary change as a result of audit	1.54	1.39	1.34	1.59	1.46
The presence of an external facilitator	2.71	2.71	2.72	2.70	2.71

DISCUSSION

Overall comparison of conventional audit and significant event auditing

Conventional audit usually requires the practice to explore a problem in some depth and to invest considerable thought and effort in its analyses. This makes it more likely that a decision or decisions to make changes, possibly quite substantial changes, in practice procedures will follow. Because of the greater investment in time, it seems possible that a decision to change, which may sometimes have been achieved quite laboriously, will be implemented, although the short duration of our study meant this could not be proven.

Significant event auditing, on the other hand, can cover a much wider range and larger number of topics for the same or even a lesser investment in time. It also appears to be less restricted in the range of areas that may be explored. The analyses, though, must of necessity be more superficial. This does not mean that this method is any less likely to promote change. Since change involves both emotional and intellectual investment, the highly emotional content of many significant event discussions may serve equally as an engine of change and the commitment to the change may even be substantially greater. The extent to which this was observed varied considerably from practice to practice and seems to have related to the extent to which the practice shared the emotional content of events or the extent of engagement with the method. Significant event auditing is of great value in scanning the range of clinical and administrative problems for those worthy of further exploration by more conventional means. It also allows the exploration of issues that might otherwise elude audit altogether. It requires, but hence engenders, greater intra-practice collaboration and team working.

Key factors associated with success in the audit process

The researchers made a number of other observations about the study practices which, while derived mainly from close involvement with them over an extended period, are broadly supported by the exit questionnaires and exit meeting. From these certain tentative conclusions could be reached regarding conditions favourable to the successful execution of audit in practices.

The role of the practice manager

It was clear from observation of the functioning of practice managers, from the comments of doctors at exit meetings, and from responses to the exit questionnaire that an enthusiastic, well trained and respected practice manager was a powerful catalyst to successful audit.

Motivation within the primary health care team

Successful practice teams appeared to be motivated by a shared vision of what they were about and by a sense of commitment to each other. Recognition of their contribution to the team effort was an important motivator of individuals, although perceived personal failure—especially if personally threatening, such as the misinterpretation of the urgency of a medical situation— was also a stimulus to personal growth and development if properly handled. Significant event auditing appeared to have more potential for this sort of individual and team motivation, though the process of audit generally does help build teamwork and mutual trust.

Team members complementary in terms of skills, functions and personal characteristics

Successful teams were often noted to include people of disparate but dove-tailing personal attributes. This appeared to make for teams that were more adaptable. A number of particular personal characteristics were felt to be more apparent in individuals in 'successful' practices including flexibility, perseverance, enthusiasm, and openness to change.

Organizational characteristics and resources

The greater resources of time, money and staff available to practices, the more likely they were to respond successfully to challenges. Adequate resourcing also seemed to boost morale. Computerization was one organizational feature consistently noted to be positively associated with success in conducting audit.

Trust, communication and team working

In well functioning teams mutual trust and respect were readily apparent. Communication flowed easily and there was a general willingness to discuss difficult and threatening issues quite openly. All team members were involved in implementing change and often in prior decision making. Appropriate delegation was also observed in successful practices.

Leadership

Leadership is a difficult issue for a general practice team which is said to be non-hierarchical and yet is often led, or apparently led, by doctors or even an individual doctor. In this study other models of leadership were observed in action and in successful practices leadership of audit activity was often seen to be shared and to move around the group in response to different challenges. The effective chairing of meetings was noted as another key to success and this too was not exclusively observed in doctors (see above under "Role of the practice manager"). Well run meetings had clear endpoints and decisions made which seemed to instil in others a commitment to take action.

Resolution of conflict

Although relations in all the study practices were generally cordial and practice business was conducted in a courteous fashion, there were times when conflict within the team was apparent. It was observed in this study that when conflict was handled constructively and intelligently it was a creative force and could stimulate useful change. In successful teams bargaining and negotiation were observed rather more than overt or even covert hostility. Humour was used in all practices to dissipate tension and defuse potential conflict.

CONCLUSIONS

Feasibility and acceptability

We have shown that the method of single case analysis for general practice which we have called significant event auditing is both feasible and acceptable in practices of various sizes in both urban and rural settings. However, it appears that to achieve success the method requires a high level of trust and good communication within the team. It probably also requires some external facilitation to begin with, although the facilitator role requires mostly generic facilitation skills combined with a good understanding of the purpose and methodology of significant event analysis as described here. It should be within the capabilities of most practices to conduct this style of audit without external assistance, although some initial help would be recommended.

Strengths and potential drawbacks

Conventional medical audit most often looks at processes in the delivery of health care. This is because of the immense, often insurmountable, difficulties in examining outcomes. Significant event analysis, while also mostly concerned with improvements to the quality of process in health care, is at least indisputably linked to outcome in its inception. Because better health outcomes are our most fundamental goal, significant event analysis has a considerable emotional appeal. Put another way, it has a high face validity. The kinds of problems identified by significant event analysis are highly practical and have a clear day-to-day relevance to the work of general practitioners. Because the process is local to the practice, in contrast to some of the more traditional forms of case-based medical audit, it provides feedback that is more immediate, comes from known peers and is delivered verbally rather than in written form. It is, in other words, the kind of feedback that has been shown to work in achieving change in the behaviour of health care professionals (Eisenberg, 1986). Furthermore, the kind of standards that emerge from significant event analysis are more likely to be practicable and workable than those that are the traditional starting point of conventional audit. The range of issues that are and may be tackled by significant event analysis is very wide and will include many of the more qualitative aspects of health care that are difficult to examine using more conventional audit methods.

One of the problems that beset much conventional audit is the generally incomplete state of medical records in general practice. While it is useful to highlight these and address them, there are some features of personal doctoring that are virtually impossible to record adequately and any effort to do so would be inefficient in terms of use of time. Significant event analysis, while still reliant on written records, can accept people's memories of events as evidence. This is justified on the grounds that events with a large emotional content are not usually forgotten and the feelings engendered will certainly be remembered very clearly. The use of such memories as data must, of course, be tempered by a recognition of the fact that memories of emotionally significant events may be subject to considerable distortions. However, even the way in which the actuality is distorted by the memories of the different people involved is itself revealing. It might be supposed that a lesser reliance on written records would make significant event analysis easier to carry out, but this is not the case. The demands of significant event analysis in terms of group interaction and trust are such that this method was not seen as any less demanding in practice, although the demands made by the two approaches to audit are distinctly different. Thus, for significant event auditing less preparatory effort was usually required of doctors but the emotional demands of some meetings and discussions were considerable. It is difficult to be categorical about what this means in terms of decision making and commitment to change. Our distinct impression gained from this study, which reinforces previous experience (Pringle, 1993), is that conventional audit, because of the investment of time and energy required for data collection, almost obliges practices to make a decision to change something—otherwise the effort appears to be wasted. However, unless there is emotional involvement, commitment to change is lacking. The study showed that while significant event analysis less often led to a suggestion for change, when a course of action or a change was decided upon, the commitment to it was considerable.

The greater reliance of significant event analysis on group interaction skills and communication, commitment and trust within the team, while making the

Table C1 Strengths and potential drawbacks of significant event auditing

Strengths
- Outcomes focused
- High emotional appeal
- High face validity
- Deals with practical and relevant issues and problems
- Deals with a wide range of issues including those otherwise difficult to quantify or audit by conventional means
- May require less preparatory effort
- Less exclusively reliant on written records
- Feedback is immediate, from known peers and verbal
- Builds trust and improves team working
- Raises interface and team issues

Potential drawbacks
- May be rather superficial
- May be threatening
- Emotionally demanding
- May require additional training to apply well
- Can expose team or interface issues that are very difficult to resolve
- Requires discipline in group discussions particularly concluding discussions with clear end points

method quite demanding, is also a strength, as the very performance of this form of audit enhances team building and engenders trust. It allows and encourages the team to celebrate their achievements in achieving quality for patients which boosts team morale. At the same time members of the team still recognize each other's vulnerability and this usually evokes greater, not less, mutual support. The requirement for good communication, trust and mutual respect do, however, make maximizing the benefits of significant event auditing more difficult in respect of people who are not directly involved. It has been highlighted how significant event analysis, because of the holistic view of problems it encourages, is likely to expose deficiencies in quality that arise at the interface between health care agencies, particularly between primary and secondary care. However, resolving these problems is quite difficult as it usually requires an approach to the other agency with a criticism about their standards. The possible resolution of this is for both to be prepared to accept the findings of each other's audits, to act on them, to liaise closely, and to work closely together on future audits.

This study has exposed some difficulties in the application of this audit method and some potential problems in its wider application. It is not, as might first appear, an easy method for general practitioners to apply. Its qualitative nature is rather unfamiliar and it demands of participants an honesty with each other and an exposure of feelings that is, at times, intensely uncomfortable. Indeed, it can become quite threatening but, as already mentioned, this is more likely to evoke concern and mutual support than to result in censure. If such enhanced team working does not flow from the introduction of the method, however, there is great danger of the performance review becoming stuck at a fairly superficial level. Without considerable discipline, and such discipline probably needs to be learnt in the presence of some external facilitator, it is easy for discussions to become too anecdotal and for inconsequential or no action to flow from them.

The strengths and potential drawbacks of significant event auditing are listed in Table C1.

Place of significant event auditing

Significant event auditing is best seen as an additional tool for the enhancement of performance review. It is complementary to and not a substitute for more conventional audit methods. It is a good screening tool for identifying problems in the quality of health care and its delivery, and in helping to set an audit agenda. Its inclusion in a practice's audit programme balances the intellectual and emotional content of performance review. Furthermore, it will extend the range of problems available to audit. By involving more of the team it helps the transition from purely medical audit (involving only doctors) to clinical audit (involving the whole primary health care team). Indeed, because nothing remains outside its reach it also encourages interface audit and opens up the possibility of joint audit with other agencies which should lead to improvements in the quality of care across interfaces—the goal of 'seamless care' comes into view. The initiation of significant event auditing in British general practice probably requires some external facilitation to begin with, and this would seem to be an ideal role for medical audit advisory groups and their audit facilitators.

RECOMMENDATIONS

First of all, we would not recommend significant event auditing as the sole method of quality assurance in general practice and would, indeed, be hesitant about practices starting with this approach to audit without first experiencing the challenges of conventional audit. This is because high levels of mutual trust and communication need to be in place before significant event analysis can successfully be carried out. To start too early with this approach could, we fear, lead to its being discredited and mean that the benefits it might bring later would be lost. For practices already on the road to quality assurance and seeking to extend their repertoire of audit skills we can recommend it. In introducing the method we would recommend that practices seek some external facilitation and we feel this ought to be provided by medical audit advisory groups. To this end we recommend that audit facilitators should be trained in significant event auditing. This is not as difficult as might first appear since many of the skills required for facilitation are more generic and to these generic skills a knowledge and understanding of significant event auditing (which this report provides) may be added. We would further recommend that practices involve all team members in significant event analysis. In particular, we would recommend that suitably trained practice managers be given a central role in the development of the method in the practice.

Finally, we would recommend that official scepticism about the value of case-based audit (SMAC, 1990), particularly in primary care, be re-examined in the light of this report and attention drawn instead to the important pre-requisites for this approach to be successfully applied and, providing these are met, encouragement and sanction be given to efforts to improve quality of care using this important additional approach.

The main purposes to which the method can usefully be applied include the selection of areas for conventional audit; extending audit into the 'softer' areas of practice activity, that is those less easily quantified but undoubtedly important; and opening up the area of interface audit. The method can also be used as a team-building tool providing there is a firm foundation to begin with.

References

Baker P (1993) The historical context of auditing and significant event auditing in particular. Speech to National Conference on Significant Event Auditing, Castle Donnington.

Balint M (1964) *The Doctor, his Patient and the Illness*. 2nd ed. Tunbridge Wells, Pitman Medical.

Baly M E (1986) *Florence Nightingale and the Nursing Legacy*. London, Croom Helm.

Barrowclough B, Bunch J and Nelson B (1974) A hundred cases of suicide: clinical aspects. *British Journal of Psychiatry* **125**, 355–73.

Bennett J and Walshe K (1990) Occurrence screening as a method of audit. *British Medical Journal* **300**, 1248–51.

Bradley C (1992) Turning anecdotes into data—the critical incident technique. *Family Practice* **9**, 98–103.

Buck N, Devlin H B and Lunn J N (1987) *The Report of a Confidential Enquiry into Peri-operative Deaths*. London, Nuffield Provincial Hospitals Trust/King's Fund.

Buckley G (1990) Clinically significant events. In Marinker M (Ed.) *Medical Audit in General Practice*. London, MSD Foundation. pp. 120–43.

Codman E A (1916) *A Study in Hospital Efficiency*. Boston, Thomas Todd Co. Cited by Donabedian E A in *Explorations in Quality Assessment and Monitoring*. Ann Arbor, Health Administration Press.

Crombie D L and Fleming D M (1988) *Practice Activity Analysis. Occasional Paper 41*. London, Royal College of General Practitioners.

Department of Health (1989) *Medical Audit. NHS Review Working Paper 6*. London, HMSO.

Department of Health (1990) Medical audit in the family practitioner services. Health Circular (FP) (90)8. London, HMSO.

Department of Health and Social Security (1986) *Report on Confidential Enquiries into Maternal Deaths in England and Wales, 1979–1980*. London, HMSO.

Donabedian A E (1982) *Explorations in Quality Assessment and Monitoring. Vol. 2: The Criteria and Standards of Quality*. Ann Arbor, Health Administration Press.

Eisenberg J M (1986) Changing physicians' practice patterns. In *Doctors' Decisions and Costs of Health Care*. Ann Arbor, Health Administration Press.

Flanagan J C (1954) The critical incident technique. *Psychological Bulletin* **51**, 327–58.

Hughes J and Humphreys C (1990) *Medical Audit in General Practice: A Practical Guide to the Literature*. London, King Edward's Hospital Fund for London.

Irvine D H (1990) Standards in general practice: the quality initiative revisited. *British Journal of General Practice* **40**, 75–77.

Lunn J N and Musher W W (1982) *Mortality Associated with Anaesthesia*. London, Nuffield Provincial Hospitals Trust.

Marinker M (1990) Principles. In Marinker M (Ed.) *Medical Audit in General Practice*. London, MSD Foundation. pp 12–13.

Medical Services Study (1978) Deaths under 50. Report to the Royal College of Physicians of London. *British Medical Journal* **2**, 1061–2.

Pendleton D, Schofield T and Marinker M (1986) *In Pursuit of Quality. Approaches to Performance Review in General Practice*. London, Royal College of General Practitioners.

Pendleton D, Schofield T, Tate P et al. (1984) *The Consultation: An Approach to Learning and Teaching*. Oxford, Oxford Medical Publications.

Pringle M (1993) *Change and Teamwork in Primary Care*. London, BMJ Books.

Pringle M, Bradley C, Carmichael C et al. (1994) A survey of attitudes to and experience of medical audit in general practice. *Audit Trends* **2**, 9–13.

Royal College of General Practitioners (1985a) *Quality in General Practice. Policy Statement 2*. London, RCGP.

Royal College of General Practitioners (1985b) *What Sort of Doctor? Assessing the Quality of Care in General Practice. Report from General Practice 23*. London, Royal College of General Practitioners.

Royal College of General Practitioners (1990) *Fellowship by Assessment. Occasional Paper 50*. London, RCGP.

Shaw C D (1980) Aspects of audit 4. *British Medical Journal* **280**, 1443–5.

Standing Medical Advisory Committee for the Secretaries of State for Health and Wales (1990) *The Quality of Medical Care*. London, HMSO.

APPENDIX 1

Significant event auditing: a user's guide

Professor Mike Pringle MD, FRGCP
Department of General Practice, Nottingham

and

Dr Colin Bradley MD, FRCGP
Senior Lecturer, Department of General Practice, Birmingham

Introduction

If we define 'medical audit' in its widest sense, the first examples are seen to be postmortems. Here all the hubris of the diagnostician was put to the test and, if the pathology was not that expected, lessons were learnt. The continuous evolution of medical knowledge through the assessment of clinical performance is the hallmark of auditing and it formed the basis of the science that we practise today.

Hospitals continued this tradition through ward rounds and case conferences. Indeed the introduction for medical students to medical audit—often unwittingly it has to be accepted—was, until recently, meetings to discuss perinatal complications. It is clear therefore that the origins of quality assurance in medicine are founded on the examination of individual cases. In nursing, by contrast, Florence Nightingale began her career by auditing the care of groups of soldiers in the Crimea, demonstrating that group audits have more political effect than case reports.

The first pressure to move away from case-based auditing in medicine occurred in the United States. In the early part of this century, a sudden influx of immigrants meant that the demand for doctors far outstripped supply. As a consequence the standards of medical attention dropped—entry to medical school without secondary education was common and the medical course consisted of two years of lectures—and then the standards of care declined.[1] Naturally this led to demands for improved standards and this resulted in the first examples of cohort auditing by doctors.[2]

Primary care entered auditing late, mainly because it was delivered for the first half of this century by singlehanded general practitioners who closely guarded their clinical freedom and who had no colleagues to undertake peer review. The advent of group practice changed this, with partners observing each other's care. Since most patients in primary care do not have florid symptoms and a quick passage to the postmortem room, it seemed most logical to look at care through group audits. This was reinforced by the wholesale transfer of the ideas of Avedis Donabedian[3,4] who had proposed the triad of structure, process and outcomes for American secondary care.

So, as British hospitals continued to refine case-based auditing into, for example, the Confidential Enquiry in Perioperative Deaths (CEPOD)[5,6,7] primary care examined workload, prescribing patterns, morbidity, patient satisfaction, referral and consultation rates.[8–14] The arrival of vocational training reinforced this image of medical audit by valuing audits of the quality of medical records, concentrating on the order and contents, not on the quality of care.

When the MAAGs were formed their visitors often entered practices to be told that no medical audit was happening. On enquiring further they would often discover that complex and effective audits had indeed been undertaken on the appointments system, prescribing, care of hypertensive patients etc, but this had not been called or recognized as 'audit'. In the same way, case-based auditing has been occurring—indeed it is the most common form of 'audit' in primary care—but has never been glorified with a name. It has therefore gone unrecognized.

It happens in corridors and over coffee. It forms the substance of anecdotes and articles. It is used in random case analysis with trainees and it is the key component of that most powerful of guardians of clinical standards—the profession's conscience. Case-based auditing is an integral part of general practice, but it is often not used effectively. A case is mentioned in passing, it is not discussed in detail, lessons are not learnt.

Significant event auditing (it started its formal life as "critical event monitoring" but that title is misleading and pejorative) is the culmination of the oldest thread in medical quality assurance and it formalizes an activity which is already part of our professional lives. It is not new in the sense of an innovation, but it is new in the sense of being fresh and it is gaining respectability—it is now a fundamental part of Fellowship by Assessment of the RCGP.[15]

What is significant event auditing?

Let us take an example. A general practitioner is called as an emergency on a Saturday afternoon to an asthmatic adult. On arrival she finds that the patient is shocked, sweaty, with a nearly silent chest. The ambulance arrives and the patient gets to hospital just in time. A life has been saved. Over coffee on Monday morning, the doctor describes how terrifying the experience was; how lucky the patient had been. The partners sympathize and get on with reading the mail.

But in a significant event auditing practice, the case will be noted down and will be discussed at a regular meeting. The partners will look at the care of this patient in a supportive way, not to allocate blame but to learn lessons. It might well want to know why the doctor was called so late in the crisis, what prophylaxis was being used, when the reviews had been undertaken and when peak flows had been recorded, whether the patient had a peak flow meter at home and if so, whether he knew when to call for advice, if the doctor had oxygen and appropriate drugs in her car, how quickly the ambulance responded, and so on.

In just such a case discussion one practice discovered that all five doctors were using radically different courses of oral steroids in acute asthma—constant dose or tailing off; 20 mg per day at the start up to 40 mg; divided doses or single doses; enteric coated or normal. If the doctors were in such disarray how could the patients be expected to 'follow medical advice'? That practice agreed a standard regime soon after and has audited it since to ensure it is being followed.

This article first appeared in *Audit Trends* (1994) **2**, 20–24 and has been reproduced by kind permission of the Editor.

This illustrates several points about significant event auditing. It is structured: there is clear purpose and a rigour in the way it is carried out. It is not an exercise in blame allocation. It reveals problems.

There are four results from the discussion of a significant event:

1. *Celebration*

Often the care given is shown to be exemplary. A patient might have mentioned lethargy at an over-75 check and the nurse arranged a full blood count which revealed the leukaemia. The event is just part of life's rich tragedy.

2. *No action*

A 45-year-old man collapses and dies from a coronary. He had been seen two years before in a well man clinic and nothing was found. He was a non-smoker. The practice could have done no more.

3. *A conventional audit*

Sometimes a problem is revealed, but the practice is unsure how common it is. After a night visit to a patient having an epileptic fit it transpires that the patient had been getting repeat prescriptions for over two years without review. Just how many patients are not attending for routine review? A conventional audit is required.

4. *Immediate change*

Some events clearly expose systematic weaknesses in the care of the practice. A patient has a stroke and the last entry in the notes reveals a very high blood pressure, but the patient did not attend for review. This is acknowledged to be both a serious and a common problem. The practice agrees to alter its recall system to allow such patients to be followed up if they fail to attend.

What is a significant event?

All the examples so far have been clinical events, but at least half are organizational. Table 1 shows a sample list which one practice uses, but every practice should decide for itself on a core list. The core list only represents those cases that should be recorded for discussion. Any other event which any team member decides is important can be recorded. It is, of course, up to any team member not to record an event because the subject is too sensitive for that person. This freedom must be respected, but happens very rarely.

Choosing events

Events should be chosen because:

- they are thought important in the life of the practice
- they may offer some insight into the general care of the practice.

If a patient leaves the practice without changing address it might be, for example, that his/her spouse is registered with another practice and they tossed a coin. It might, however, mean that at least one patient finds the appointment system and attitude of a receptionist unacceptable. How many other potential emigrés might there be out there? One practice writes a routine letter to all such patients asking for their honest comments and the replies are taken to the significant event meeting.

Table 1 A possible initial list of significant events

Preventive care:	Whooping cough
	Measles
	Mumps
	Unplanned pregnancy
	A pregnancy with no clear recording of rubella immunization/immunity
	Positive cervical smear
	Non-accidental injury
	Orchidopexy
	Congenital dislocation of hip
	Hearing aid (under 12)
	Squint diagnosed by ophthalmologist
	Diagnosis of tuberculosis
	Abnormal liver function tests (alcohol)
Acute care:	Sudden unexpected death
	Myocardial infarction
	Cerebrovascular accident
	Suicidal attempt
	All new cancer diagnoses
	Renal failure
	Intra-uterine or perinatal death
	Sudden Infant Death Syndrome
Chronic disease:	Diabetes: registered partially sighted/blind
	Urgent visit for diabetic problem
	Diagnosis of MI, CVA or TIA
	Leg ulcer or amputation
	Asthma: urgent visit request, hospital admissions
	Epilepsy: status epilepticus
Organization:	Home visit accepted but not done
	Letter received but not acted upon
	Abnormal path results (e.g. smear) not acted upon
	A breach of confidentiality
	Patient changes practice without changing address
	Complaint about the appointment system
	Urgent appointment request not seen in 12 hours
	Routine appointment (any doctor) not available for more than 2 working days
	Routine appointment for a specific doctor not available for more than 3 working days
	Referral letter not sent
	Any patient complaint
	Upset staff

How does a practice do significant event auditing?

The first essential is for the practice to have mature relationships and to be confident that interpersonal problems will not be exacerbated by frank discussion. In our study we found that most practices fulfilled this criterion.

The second requirement is that the practice team—start perhaps with doctors, nurses and managers and then include receptionists etc—is prepared to put aside time. One hour every two months is all that is required and this is usually possible within even the busiest of practices.

It is very helpful if one member of the team is prepared to act as the leader for this activity—reminding people to record significant events, ensuring the meetings are remembered, and so on. Some practices use an external facilitator for the meetings. If you have a practice counsellor or someone similar, then ask them to chair the meetings. The team needs to appoint a secretary to the meeting who will ensure that all the lists and notes are present and that decisions are recorded.

Next the practice needs to agree a list of core events which will be routinely discussed (Table 1). Usually this list is on the reverse of the event entry sheets which are kept on every doctor's desk, in the treatment room, on the front desk and in the manager's office.

At the start of each meeting, the team quickly runs through the decisions from the last meeting and checks that actions agreed are being carried out. Next each person is asked in turn to select one of their events for discussion. Each person gets a chance to present a case in turn around the room until everybody has had one chance. The team can start a second round.

Obviously some team members might choose 'safe' cases, but as confidence in colleagues increases, team members increasingly offer those that might seem less straightforward. A well developed team will offer everybody the space to allow their confidence to grow.

After each case discussion one of the four types of decisions are arrived at and recorded. Where action is agreed, one person is identified as responsible for carrying out that action.

Why bother?

No practice is going to go to all the effort of setting up significant event auditing if it does not get something out of it. The following reasons can be put forward:

1. *It is enjoyable*

General practitioners have always enjoyed sharing clinical experience, swapping stories and marvelling at the complexity of human nature. Well, significant events meetings offer that in aces.

2. *It is challenging*

While conventional group-based audits are intellectually challenging, significant event auditing is both emotionally and intellectually demanding. It stretches assumptions and complacencies more powerfully than other audit methods.

3. *It complements other quality activity*

Conventional audits are best carried out in an area which the practice perceives to be a concern. Significant event auditing identifies those concerns and offers guidance as to where conventional audits might be most fruitful.

4. *It can be a real change*

There is a tendency to react to conventional audits with platitudes, but for nothing really to change: "Yes I'll try to remember to look at the fundi of more diabetics". But a significant event in which a diabetic goes blind because her retinopathy was not detected provokes a real change. It appeals to the heart, and change is an emotional experience.

But a word of caution. One significant event does not herald a heatwave or a nuclear winter: if one case has been handled excellently, it does not mean that all are: if one was a disaster, many others may be exemplary. Each case needs to be kept in proportion and decisions need to be mature and logical.

The role of the MAAG

Some practices have started significant event auditing without help or prompting. For many others, however, it needs stimulation. The MAAG's roles can be:

1. To inform practices that significant event auditing is one of their audit options
2. To train general practitioners, nurses and managers in the technique at meetings and seminars
3. To offer facilitation for the early meetings
4. To bring practices together so that they can share their experience of significant event auditing and expand their skills.

Conclusion

The pursuit of quality is a cultural endeavour. It has no fixed methods, no pre-conceived outcomes. Practices need to experiment with many ways of auditing in order to keep their quality initiatives alive. Significant event auditing offers one such option.

Significant event auditing cannot, however, replace conventional auditing. It complements it by exploring the age old skills of case-based auditing and linking it into the newer concept of group audits. A quality practice will want to do both. Significant event auditing has a power that is out of all proportion to the work involved. It has great potential to engender real change in the practice.

References

1. Lembcke PA (1967) Evaluation of medical audit. *Journal of the American Medical Association* **199**, 543–550.
2. Flexner A (1910) *Medical Evaluation in United States and Canada*. Report to the Carnegie Foundation. New York, Merrymount Press.
3. Donabedian A (1985) The methods and findings of quality assessment and monitoring—an illustrative analysis. In *Explorations in Quality Assurance and Medical Malpractice*. Michigan, Health Administration Press.
4. Donabedian A (1966) Evaluating the quality of medical care. *Milbank Memorial Fund Quarterly* **44**, 166–204.
5. Heath DA (1990) Random review of hospital patients' records. *British Medical Journal* **300**, 651–2.
6. Buck N, Devlin HB and Lunn JN (1987) *The Report of a Confidential Enquiry into Perioperative Deaths*. London, Nuffield Provincial Hospitals Trust and King Edward's Hospital Fund for London.
7. Hopkins A (1991) Approaches to medical audit. *Journal of Epidemiology and Community Health* **45**, 1–3.
8. Curtis P (1974) Medial audit in general practice. *Journal of the Royal College of General Practitioners* **24**, 607–11.
9. Forsyth G and Logan RLF (1962) Studies in medical care. In *Towards a Measure of Medical Care*. Oxford, OUP.
10. Cartwright A (1967) *Patients and Their Doctors. A Study in General Practice*. London, Routledge & Kegan Paul.
11. Seiler ER (1967) Immunisation in general practice—analysis of some of the factors involved. *Journal of the Royal College of General Practitioners* **13**, 197–204.
12. Korsch BM, Gozzi EK and Francis V (1968) Gaps in doctor-patient communication. 1. Doctor-patient interaction and satisfaction. *Paediatrics* **42**, 855–71.
13. Drury M and Kuenssberg EV (1970) Inquiry into administrative activities in general practice. *British Medical Journal* **4**, 42–44.
14. Honigsbaum F (1972) Quality in general practice—a commentary on the quality of care provided by general practitioners. *Journal of the Royal College of General Practitioners* **22**, 429–51.
15. Royal College of General Practitioners (1990) *Fellowship by Assessment*. Occasional Paper 50. London, RCGP.

APPENDIX 2

All significant events listed for possible discussion at significant events meetings

Notes:

1. Those significant events actually discussed are highlighted [in italics], and the numbers to their left indicate the case numbers in Appendix 3 (Clinical) and Appendix 4 (Administrative).

2. For events which were listed on multiple occasions, the number of such listings is given in brackets after the significant event.

A. CLINICAL

1. Cancers and tumours

1	*Carcinoma of the larynx*
2–6	*Carcinoma of the bronchus* (13)
7–11	*Carcinoma of the breast* (8)
12	*A group of 5 new diagnoses of breast cancer*
13–14	*Cancer of the body of uterus* (5)
15	*Squamous carcinoma of the vulva*
16	*Ovarian cyst* (2)
17	*Brain tumour* (5)
	Spinal tumour
	Renal carcinoma (2)
18–19	*Bladder tumour* (2)
20	*Cancer of the prostate* (6)
21	*Carcinoma of the oesophagus*
	Carcinoma of the stomach (5)
22	*Duodenal tumour*
23	*Liver secondaries*
24	*Carcinoma of the colon* (7)
	Rectal carcinoma (2)
25	*Parathyroid tumour*
26	*Leukaemia* (6)
27	*Multiple myeloma* (2)
28	*Lymphoma*
	Malignant lymph nodes
	Basal cell carcinoma (2)
	Intra-epidermal skin cancer (2)
29–30	*Pelvic mass* (2)
	Carcinomatosis (2)
31	*Five new diagnoses of cancer*
32	*Testicular tumour*

2. Contraception, obstetrics, and gynaecology

33–34	*Injectable contraception* (2)
35	*Postcoital contraception*
36	*Oral contraception*
37–38	*Unplanned pregnancy* (28)
	Pregnant with IUCD (2)
	Termination request
39	*Termination at 24 weeks for medical reasons*
40	*Fetal abnormality on ultrasound scan*
	No fetal heart heard at 18 weeks
	Ectopic pregnancy (3)
41	*No evidence of rubella immunity at confirmation of pregnancy* (4)
42	*Miscarriage* (3)
	Stillbirth of twins
43–44	*Home delivery request* (3)
	Postnatal visits
45	*Oestradiol implant*
	Hormone replacement therapy (2)

46–47	*Abnormal smear* (3)
	Overdue for smear test

3. Sudden deaths, cardiovascular and cerebrovascular accidents

48–65	*Sudden death* (44)
	Cardiac arrest
66–75	*Myocardial infarction* (47)
	Death following angioplasty
	Ruptured aortic aneurysm (2)
	Angina (4)
	Abnormal ECG—aged 6
	Paroxysmal SVT (2)
	Intermittent heart block
	Sick sinus syndrome
	Congestive cardiac failure
	Collapse—?Stokes-Adams
76–78	*Pulmonary embolus* (6)
79	*Deep vein thrombosis* (3)
80–88	*Cerebrovascular accident* (17)

4. The major chronic diseases including diabetes mellitus

89	*Hypertension*
	Hypertension—failure of follow-up
90–93	*Diabetes mellitus, diagnosis* (12)
	Diabetes mellitus, admission (1)
94–103	*Diabetes mellitus, complication* (28)
104–106	*Diabetic—poor control* (4)
	No diabetic review (4)
107–111	*Epilepsy* (9)
	Sudden collapse with probable convulsion
112	*Multiple sclerosis* (2)
	Hydrocephalus
	Acute confusional state
113–125	*Acute exacerbation of asthma* (27)
	Thyrotoxicosis
	Hypothyroid

5. Paediatrics

126	*Non-accidental injury* (2)
127	*Congenital dislocation of the hip*
128	*Undescended testicle* (2)
	Neonatal obstruction
	Paediatric admission
	Child abuse examination—no warning

6. Gastro-intestinal and renal

	Abdominal pain (2)
	Acute appendicitis
	Subacute bowel obstruction

19   *Abuse to district nurse*
      Patient would not see locum
      The right not to treat unco-operative patients
20   *Request for oral contraception during son's appointment*
      Intoxicated person walks into surgery
      Medication under false pretences
      Three members of family in A & E in 1 week
      Aggressive manner at well-man clinic
21   *Anger about wife changing daughter's name*
      Threatening behaviour in surgery

3. Prescribing and dispensing

22–25 *Dispensing errors (dispensing practices)* (15)
      Wrong dose of drug dispensed by local pharmacy
      Non-delivery of urgent tablets
      Vaccinations left out of fridge for 24 hours
26   *Prescription tampered with* (3)
27   *Prescription request by telephone*
      Change in strength of tablets
28   *Hib given instead of flu vaccination*
29   *Flu vaccine given instead of tetanus*
30   *Meningitis vaccine*
      80 flu vaccinations left
      Repeat prescriptions
      No pain relief
31   *Efcortelan out of date in nurses' room*
32   *Resistance to erythromycin*

4. Breaches of policies or protocols or procedures

33   *New heart attack protocol*
      Issue of nebulizer protocol
      Telephone protocol
34   *Practice policy on appointment system*
      Practice policy on cholesterol tests and advice
      Asthma audit
      Hypothyroid audit
      Audit in general
35   *Digoxin audit*
      Nurse protocol query
36   *At-risk groups—protocol*
      Urines—routine testing
      Giving doctors' home telephone numbers
      New patients 52–55—to be included in current breast
      screening programme
37–38 *Elderly patients at risk*

5. Home visits, emergencies and out-of-hours problems

39   *Visit not done* (5)
      Emergency call outside practice area
      No reply received when patient rang surgery in
      evening
      Nursing home visit request
      Answering service fault
40   *Accident call-out—severe disruption to surgery*
      Unable to page doctor on call (2)
      Difficulty in obtaining district nurse
41   *Phone not properly transferred*
      Three urgent calls phoned in in two minutes
      Early call-out—?policy
      8 a.m. morning call
      Medical review slip created unnecessary visit
      Reception not notified when urgent call out occurs
      Unable to locate oxygen and other emergency
      equipment
      Long-term visit: administration

6. Premises

      Dispensary door not locked after evening surgery

Burglar alarm triggered (4)
Front door not locked properly
Premises insecure 1.30 a.m.
42   *Branch surgery in connection with improvements*
43   *Surgery building*
44   *Blanket burn from lamp*
      Power cut
      Fault on fire board
      Drains blocked
      Saturday morning nurses' room
      Medication review
      Downstairs room—no equipment
      Anglepoise lamp came apart during smear
      Telephone fault
      Nebulizer in nurses' room not complete

7. Rota

      Staff not informed of change of duty doctor
      Days off
45   *Trainee on duty alone* (2)
46   *Only two doctors working—one called out*
47   *Two rota changes leaving only one doctor on*
48   *Rota changes*
      Antenatal clinic not cancelled—doctor on leave
      No half days in week
      11.30 a.m. surgery—1 out of 4 doctors
      Only one doctor available noon–7 p.m.

8. Meetings

      Meeting with community health council
      Inquest availability
49   *Case conference—at-risk register*
50   *HRT talk—no nurse present*
      Asthma meeting—partner away

9. Personnel

      Staff upsets (8)
      Staff holidays
      Receptionist gives notice
      One receptionist short Monday morning
      Row with district nurse
      Appointment of senior receptionist
      Staff appraisal
      Decision to dismiss member of staff

10. Communication within primary health care team

51   *Lack of liaison between health care professionals*
52   *Failure of communication—nurses*
      Communication failure over results of tests

11. Confidentiality

      Discussion between doctors and nurses in reception
53–55 *Confidential information leak* (4)
      Father seeks confirmation of appointments

12. Secondary care

      Surgical admission to hospital closed
56   *Sudden collapse—999 call—no ambulance*
57   *Hospital discharge without instructions*
      Hospital communication—wife very upset
      Patient angry about referral
      Transport for DXT
58   *Hospital admission slip lost*
      Letter about DNA hospital appointment

59 *Letter sent appointment not received*
No female geriatric beds available at usual hospitals

60 *Supply of tablets kept by hospital on discharge* (2)
Letter from public health about hepatitis A 2 weeks after notification
Patient to telephone consultant
Discharge letter
Delay in smear processing 6 or 7 weeks
Eye appointment
Delayed admission

61 *Late arrival of ambulance to emergency call*

13. Errors of omission

Meals on wheels referral not made
Forgot to write prescription (2)

62 *Pathology specimens not delivered to hospital*

63 *Patient not informed of change of medication* (2)

64–66 *Missed referral* (9)

67 *Patient request for sight of report before posting—system failed*

68 *Letter to reduce medication not acted on*

69 *No letter after smear test* (2)

70 *No death certificate available for relatives*

71 *Second private certificate—first not charged*
Cremation form not completed
No doctor at surgery at appointed time Sunday
Daytime visit request but nothing written in day book
Tetanus missed at new patient clinic

72 *Letter not written for urgent appointment*

73–74 *Report received, not acted on* (6)

75 *Note attached to patient's notes, but not responded to* (2)

76 *Name changed on computer, but not on records* (2)

77 *Discharge not on computer*

14. Errors of commission

Letters delivered in error to another surgery
Insurance form error (2)

78 *Nebulizer issued without patient being seen*

79 *Poor patient/doctor communication about blood tests*

80 *Wrong information given over telephone about results*

81 *New patient allocated to wrong doctor*

82 *Positive smear result given to patient as negative*

15. Appointments

Small attendance at surgery
Nurse gone home. Patient in waiting room $1\frac{1}{2}$ hrs

83 *Patient in waiting room 2 hours*
RAF patients—attendances

84 *Failure of patients to attend clinic*
Grouping of appointments in relation to health promotion clinics
Minor operations—nurse assistance
Wart clinic running late
Double booked minor operation
DNA appointments—20 minutes × 2

85–86 *Appointment system* (21)
ECG urgent request—no appointments available
Very long consultation during surgery—patients angry
Unannounced extra patient
Employer will not allow time to see doctor
Two interruptions to borrow and return ophthalmoscope
'Lost' patient—sat for 30 minutes—no notes
Patient arrived for foreign travel clinic at 8.10 a.m.
Patient arrived 1 hour early—given first appointment

87 *Emergency treatment—nursing appointments full*
Patient discussed marital difficulties in appointment for baby's nappy rash
Father requested hay fever medication at daughter's appointment
1.15 p.m. appointment—premises locked
Patient attended—no notes, no warning
Four patients added on end of surgery—attended in middle
Failed appointment
DNA new patient medical
Surgery cancelled—patient not informed

16. Contractual issues

88–89 *Failure to meet immunization target* (2)

17. Administration

90 *Non-identification of patient*
Default for preschool check not detected
Computer problem (10)

91 *Installation of new computer*

92 *Financial problem* (2)

93 *Practice progress*
Tetanus booster response to letter/reminder

94 *Patient had three inappropriate letters*
Unnecessary recall letters sent before summary updated on computer
Recall letter inappropriate (patient pregnant)
In practice one year—not signed on
Patients with similar names

95 *Not 'our' patient*
Two 'same name' patients—wrong notes
FHSA notification of deaths
Nursing home death registration
Return of Standard Life form
Temporary resident forms not being signed
Death slips not going to secretary
Confusion over change of address
Collection box cleared too early
Patient not on list

96–99 *No seats available in waiting room* (9)

18. Medical records

100–103 *Notes misfiled* (4)
No record of consultation in notes
Notes unavailable for consultation (4)
No record of diabetic check
No record of visit

104 *Thyroid function test result not on computer*
Ampicillin prescription not entered on computer
Inhaler prescribed—nothing in notes or on computer
Smear date incorrect on computer
No notes available baby immunization clinic
Temporary resident form—no details
FP1001 tag in notes aged 7

105 *Wrong address on notes* (2)

19. Patient information and services

106 *Information requested on AIDS in reception*
Patients' transport services

20. Training and continuing education

FHSA training—clinics etc.

107 *Surfeit of training*
New staff member training

21. Legal issues

22. Other

APPENDIX 3

Clinical significant events discussed in audit meetings

1. New cancer diagnosis: larynx

Presented with sore throat, slight dysphagia, weight loss. ? viral illness treated with paracetamol. One month later, sore throat persisting, feeling poorly. Weight down five pounds. Treated with antibiotics. Refer if comes back. A few weeks later, pains in face, earache, husky voice. Antibiotics prescribed. Urgent ear, nose and throat appointment. Patient seen privately for barium swallow and pharyngoscopy. Diagnosis made and x-ray therapy given. Picked up fairly quickly.

Discussion: Continuity of care.

Decision: Encourage continuity of care.

2. New cancer diagnosis: treated for vulval problems but had carcinoma of the bronchus

Patient suffered with severe vulval problems and had a past history of tuberculosis and chronic obstructive airways disease. Sent for vulval biopsy but cancelled. Patient sore and anxious. Two weeks later, huge weight loss and thought to be possibly a malignancy of the vulva. Diagnosis Ca bronchus. Previous chest x-ray had revealed nothing abnormal.

Discussion: Surprise at diagnosis in view of symptoms presented.

Decision: Nothing to be done but try not to be blinkered by one particular symptom.

3. New cancer diagnosis in a non-insulin dependent diabetic patient

Patient presented not feeling well and complaining of a dry cough. X-ray revealed a shadow. Bronchoscopy normal, CT scan equivocal. Mediastinoscopy revealed bronchial cancer. No histology to date. This patient was a poorly complying diabetic, reluctant to take oral preparations. His weight loss was attributed to compliance with advice. He is a white-collar worker, spouse non-smoker, no industrial exposure, and non-smoker himself. Now on steroids for ? brain secondaries and bone pain.

Discussion: As above.

Decision: Nothing to be done. All care given.

4. Newly diagnosed bronchial carcinoma

Previous history of bronchitis and tuberculosis. Carcinoma not picked up on x-ray, probably because of cavitation from old tuberculosis lesion. Full blood count showed a raised plasma viscosity and repeat chest x-ray showed a carcinogenic right lung.

Discussion: As above.

Decision: Nothing to be done.

5. Squamous cell carcinoma of the lung

Presented with breathlessness and chest pain. Referred.

Discussion: Patient picked up and referred at first presentation.

Decisions: (a) To monitor all new cancer diagnoses for time taken to refer to hospital, time taken to get hospital consultation, and time taken to receive definitive treatment. (b) To place all newly diagnosed cancer patients on a monitoring list.

6. New cancer diagnosis: small cell lung

Presented with bronchospasm. Treated with Bricanyl and Pulmicort turbohaler. No better and treated with oral steroids. Previous history of bronchitis. Chest x-ray to exclude left ventricular failure revealed heart enlarged and inflammatory changes. Treated with antibiotics. Seen again with dyspnoea + +. Admitted. ? bronchospasm, treated with steroids. Improved and went on holiday. Back to clinic after holidays, found to have cervical nodes. Investigated, diagnosed, treated with chemotherapy.

Discussion: Clues to diagnosis may have been found in pain, which may have made for earlier diagnosis but it was thought that six weeks from presenting to definitive treatment was reasonable in view of the fact that the tumour did not show up on x-ray and this patient had received hospital treatment.

Decision: No decision.

7. Recurrent carcinoma of the breast: treated with topical oestrogens for atrophic vaginitis

Left-sided mastectomy in 1970s—poor prognosis. 1980s treated for atrophic vaginitis. Treatment discontinued after 3 years. Now presented with pain in right upper quadrant, which was diagnosed as secondary growths from original growth 14 years previously.

Discussion: Controversies surrounding the prescribing of topical oestrogens to patients who have had a previous malignancy.

Decision: Possibly to offer patients on topical oestrogens progesterone at yearly intervals.

8. New cancer diagnosis: 12 months after clear mammogram

Patient presented one year ago complaining her right arm thicker than left. Clinically nothing found. Referred. Mammogram nothing found. Twelve months later at breast screening, cancer found in upper inner quadrant. No axillary nodes. Consultants said this was not related to the arm swelling.

Discussion: As above.

Decision: Nothing to be done.

9. Breast lump: new cancer diagnosis

New patient with new baby went to previous practice for postnatal examination. No lump found. Came to practice for contraceptive advice, breasts not examined. Two weeks later discovered a lump, seen in two days, needle biopsy, lumpectomy, x-ray therapy.

Discussion: Reluctance of women to have their breasts examined.

Decision: To examine the breasts of all patients who present for postnatal examination.

10. New cancer diagnosis: breast

Malignant lump removed from breast. There were no nodes but as the lump was attached to deep tissue it was decided to give the patient x-ray therapy.

Discussion: The possible result of a deficiency in care for women. Breast screening not yet available. It was generally agreed that there are no factors for modifying risk. Women are extremely reluctant to have their breasts examined.

Decision: No decision.

11. New cancer diagnosis: breast

Seen at breast screening clinic having had breasts examined one month previously. Leaflets given on breast examination. Follow-up one month later. Lesion in right breast aspirated for cytology. Showed malignant cells in keeping with mammogram. Treatment wide local excision biopsy with axillary clearance, plus x-ray therapy and tamoxifen. No family history.

Discussion: Agreed it was worth sending patients for breast screening.

Decision: No decision.

12. Five new cases of carcinoma of breast discussed under one heading

(a) Patient aged 98 presented with breast lump, treated with tamoxifen.
(b) Patient presented with large breast lump referred to surgeons for excision, treatment to be decided.
(c) One-week history of breast lump referred to surgeons, treatment to be decided.
(d) *In situ* carcinoma breast, local biopsy, grade 1 carcinoma for mastectomy.
(e) Mammography revealed *in situ* changes, biopsy revealed grade 2 carcinoma. Patient had recent hormone replacement implant.

Discussion: As above.

Decision: Nothing to be done.

13. Adenocarcinoma uterus

Patient aged 60, recently married, presented with post-menopausal bleeding (PMB). Referred. Further bleeding. Re-referred for D&C. Hysterectomy subsequently performed on diagnosis. Patient not told.

Discussion: Disquiet that referral did not follow normal route and consultant's attitude to PMB investigation. Expected D&C and further investigation at first referral. Difficulty felt with patient unaware of diagnosis.

Decision: To telephone consultant before six-week follow-up, to discuss matter with husband and always to investigate postmenopausal bleeding.

14. Pre-endometrial carcinoma

Menopausal symptoms for many years. Discussed and advised about hormone replacement therapy and risks with unopposed oestrogen treatment. Referred. Various treatments tried were unacceptable as were regular D&Cs. Patient difficult to advise and took treatment into own hands despite frequent warnings.

Discussion: Problems of unopposed oestrogen therapy. The need to keep copious notes and letters for the future.

Decision: No decision.

15. Squamous carcinoma vulva

Patient aged 40 had subarachnoid haemorrhage some time ago. Hemiplegic, epileptic and wheelchair bound. Long history of genital ulcers thought to be herpes. Presented with vaginal discharge and sore on labia. Treated. Did not improve and referred. Cancer of the vulva excised within 3 weeks.

Discussion: A possible original misdiagnosis of herpes or a precursor to cancerous state. Genetic susceptibility (grandmother had radical vulvectomy). Partner congratulated on speed with which condition dealt with.

Decision: No decision.

16. Ovarian cyst

Patient aged 74 presented with ankle swelling and abdominal distension. One leg larger than other. Pelvic examination revealed large mass. Diagnosis benign ovarian tumour.

Discussion: The value of rectal and vaginal examinations in diagnosis. Leg oedema as a symptom of lower abdominal causes.

Decision: A pelvic examination to be done to consider abdominal causes when a patient presents with leg oedema.

17. Glioma

Young woman with rapid onset of glioma. Presented with two-week history of headache. Became confused. Admitted and died within a few days.

Discussion: Diagnosis with CT scan. Possible treatment if diagnosed earlier but very subtle in approach.

Decision: No decision.

18. Bladder tumour

Female patient aged 70 collapsed and complained of feeling faint. Admitted. Atrial fibrillation. Treated with drugs. Returned after 4 months with frequency and dysuria. Midstream specimen of urine positive. Treated. Several repeat midstream urine checks positive and treated with antibiotics. Midstream urine positive again four months later. Intravenous pyelogram showed bladder tumour. Referred.

Discussion: Earlier intravenous pyelogram for recurrent urinary tract infection or referral for cytoscopy. Possibility of connection between tumours and atrial fibrillation.

Decision: To take recurrent urinary tract infections seriously in elderly patients.

19. Intravenous pyelogram revealed a filling defect: probably carcinoma bladder

Patient a diabetic monitored regularly for many years.

Discussion: As above.

Decision: Place on monitoring list.

20. Carcinoma of the prostate

69-year-old man presented with low back pain. Treated for back strain. Saw osteopath. Worsening pain, sweating and anorexia. Saw partner again one month later. X-ray normal. Prostate feels normal but increasing pain and not responding to drugs. Referred for prostatic biopsy.

Discussion: Length of time to establish diagnosis.

Decision: No decision.

21. New cancer diagnosis: carcinoma of the oesophagus

Patient is late middle-aged ex-smoker who has been treated over the past year for vascular disease. Also troubled with an hiatus hernia which was diagnosed six years before. Drinks six units of alcohol per week. Presented with dysphagia and pain. Prescribed cimetidine and referred. Malignancy found on endoscopy. Oesophagus resectioned.

Discussion: The importance of referring middle-aged patients even though the thinking is that hiatus hernia should be treated by general practitioners.

Decision: No decision.

22. Duodenal tumour

29-year-old woman presented with nausea and gastric pain. Treated cimetidine. Returned with loss of weight and heartburn. Stressed. Haemoglobin 10.7. Treated Zantac and iron. Returned with abdominal pain left iliac fossa and diarrhoea. Nothing felt abdominally. Repeat haemoglobin and erythrocyte sedimentation rate—normal. Referred. Endoscopy confirmed duodenal mass. Biopsy malignant. Pancreas removed.

Discussion: Delay in diagnosis possibly due to seeing different doctors at surgery and presenting with different symptoms. Tumour not expected. Psychological aspect of patient caring for ill relative. Stage at which to initiate investigations.

Decisions: To be more aware. To instigate investigations if symptoms return before course of treatment finished and to consider barium meal at second presentation of such symptoms.

23. Carcinoma of the liver

Woman aged 29 presented for postnatal check. Returned two months later with pyrexia, vomiting, urine frequency and diarrhoea. Large lump felt. Liver function tests elevated. Partner requested liver scan. Refused. Referred and seen in 2 weeks. Liver scan showed liver adenoma due to contraceptive pill and did not require biopsy. Biopsy eventually done 4 months later. Diagnosis cancer. Treated chemotherapy.

Discussion: Unusual diagnosis for age and odd presentation. Partner unhappy about refusal of liver scan and late biopsy. Site of primary tumour.

Decision: To consider possibility of malignancy whatever age of patient and to request future scans at a different hospital if refused at first.

24. Carcinoma of the bowel: barium enema negative

Woman aged 56 presented with rectal bleeding. Barium enema negative—a little diverticular disease but no colonic abnormality. Further episodes of fresh bleeding. Colonoscopy was performed confirming diagnosis with liver metastases. Mother had died of cancer of colon.

Discussion: Rectal bleeding and occult blood tests in early diagnosis of bowel cancer. Unreliability of barium enema and necessity of further testing. Local interest in screening programme being set up. Awareness of AIDS when doing tests. Possibility of gaining skills in sigmoidoscopy.

Decision: To refer to gastro-enterologist for further testing after barium enema when patient presents with rectal bleeding and partner to collect more information on setting up screening programme in practice clinic.

25. Delay in diagnosis: parathyroid tumour

Presented three times with urinary symptoms. Blood tests not done for 5 months. Mild anaemia and mild renal failure.

Hypercalcaemic. Referred. Patient admitted for surgery. Sent home for stabilizing when high blood pressure discovered by surgeon. Further 6 weeks to wait with symptoms worsening.

Discussion: Blood pressure possibly done but not noted or acted upon and the need particularly to check pressures with renal and hyperthyroid cases. Hypertensive drug therapy.

Decision: To check blood pressures more often.

26. Chronic lymphatic leukaemia

Raised white cell count of 16 000. Referred. Had regular blood tests over several years with count gradually increasing. Last normal count ten years before at 6500.

Discussion: At what blood count level should action be taken?

Decision: To check laboratory threshold and to question any result over 12 000.

27. Carcinoma of the prostate

Elderly man with osteo-arthritis and pain in back. Lives alone. Analgesics given. Eventual erythrocyte sedimentation rate done (142) and haemoglobin (8.6). Admitted. Diagnosis carcinoma prostate with secondaries. On hormone treatment. Pain now gone.

Discussion: Problem ignored. Felt practice had colluded with daughter to keep comfortable and nothing more. Need for carers to know diagnosis. Unable to contact relatives when needed to admit.

Decision: Never to ignore back pain and to continue blood tests until diagnosis clear.

28. Delay in diagnosis: advanced lymphoma

Female patient aged 57 presented with very vague abdominal symptoms. Leg swelling which settled. Blood tests normal. Nothing on examination. Later developed abdominal swelling. Referred. Not seen immediately—no apparent urgency. Barium enema normal. Returned feeling ill. Blood tests repeated and raised. Urgent tests requested after delay of 2/3 months from initial presentation.

Discussion: Original blood test results and falsely reassured by negative barium enema result. Vague presentation by patient. Length of time taken by hospital to do tests.

Decision: Not to be reassured by blood test results, to stick by gut feeling and to push for further tests if not sure.

29. Missed pelvic mass

Female patient presented with abdominal pain, flatulence, backache and spinal stiffness. Examined—? irritable bowel syndrome. Further rectal examination 5 days later—? diverticulitis. Referred. Large pelvic mass found.

Discussion: Non-discovery of mass at rectal examination and need for vaginal examination. Treatment—everything possible done correctly. Clue felt to be in back pain.

Decision: No decision.

30. Pelvic mass

Female patient aged 50 presented with tiredness. Later consulted another partner with very heavy period and pain—? menopausal symptoms. Not examined at this time. Telephoned later—in bed, unwell and still bleeding. Partner examined and found tender smooth mass in pelvis, separate from uterus. Ectopic pregnancy excluded. Abscess diagnosed.

Treated with antibiotics. Partner examined 3 days later—no better. Told partner a coil *in situ* since 1970s. Patient admitted for hysterectomy. Following discharge, patient presented with pain top left leg into groin. No swelling or discolouration—? pelvic infection. Treated amoxycillin. Venogram. Thrombosis diagnosed.

Discussion: Vaginal examination in first instance despite patient's reluctance. Delay in hospitalization given symptoms of raised white blood count/tender/unwell. Recent hot flushes treated with Mercilon. Length of time coil *in situ*. Letter received late 1980s recommending removal. Patient declined. Anticoagulation with heparin of hysterectomy patients. Hormone replacement therapy in thrombosis patients after ovarian hysterectomy.

Decision: Act on blood results at earliest opportunity. Admit patients with pelvic mass at earliest opportunity and ask whether patient has coil *in situ*, what type and for how long.

31. Five new neoplasms: 2 carcinoma bladder, intestinal lymphoma, carcinoma testicle, carcinoma lung

It was decided to look at these patients as a group and monitor how long it took them to be referred, how long it took for them to see a consultant and how long it took for them to get treatment.

Discussion: It would appear that even though patients are being referred quickly by general practitioners, it is taking a long time to get appointments at specialist centres and a long time to receive treatment.

Decision: It was thought that by monitoring waiting times it would be possible to use the results as ammunition when pressing for appointments.

32. Simple hydrocele turned out to be malignant tumour

Patient presented with an apparently simple hydrocele. Delay before surgery. At operation, a teratoma was found and the patient's testicle removed.

Discussion: As above.

Decision: Place on monitoring list.

33. Injectable contraception: refusal of examination

New patient seen by locum requesting contraception. Would not take Pill. Disadvantages explained and personality problem noted. Given Depo-Provera. Subsequently seen by appointment by partner. Drug not available at time due to bad communication on patient's part with reception and patient very aggressive. Other possible treatments and risks attached to requested treatment explained but nothing suitable. Patient refused smear test and partner declined to give drug. Patient left very angry and not returned. Patient considered capable of giving informed consent.

Discussion: Necessity of vaginal examinations and smear tests. Flexibility needed and communication with patient in difficult cases. Use of injectable contraceptive drugs and the precedent set in this case by presence of locum.

Decision: Clinical decisions to be made according to circumstances. A disclaimer to be used in difficult cases accepting that a vaginal examination has been offered but refused. Depo-Provera has a place in certain situations and a degree of flexibility needed when dealing with difficult patients.

34. Increase in number of patients being given Depo-Provera

One partner uses quite often. Others more reticent.

Discussion: Patients to whom prescribed. Convenience factor and other uses. Financial costs as against the contraceptive pill. Nurse time involved. Timing of injections. Possible adverse reactions and difficulty of reversing.

Decision: Small audit to be undertaken to determine number of patients involved and any difficulties arising.

35. Prescribing of PC4

Patient seen on 72-hour limit. Time wasted owing to patient unable to tell reception staff reason for urgency. Partner happy to prescribe immediately to relieve possible distress and counsel at an appropriate appointment later. Other partners said would prefer to see first.

Discussion: Possible complications from drug and necessity to see patient before prescribing. Privacy factor when telephoning for urgent appointment of this nature and perhaps talk to practice manager when doctor not available. Uniform policy: worry voiced as to whether patient would return for consultation following prescribing. To educate patients as to service available by putting up publicity notice.

Decision: To see patient at earliest opportunity before prescribing. To approach drug company as to possible sign advertising service.

36. New patient request for repeat prescription: Eugynon 30

Partner involved away. Other partners felt they would give temporary repeat until notes available. Not felt to be a problem if patient on list.

Discussion: Practice formulary and new protocol being worked out.

Decision: Nothing further at this time.

37. Unplanned pregnancy

Patient aged 21 requested termination with complete confidentiality. Referred and offered immediate appointment. Practice asked to inform patient. Termination completed and postoperative follow-up at practice well woman clinic.

Discussion: Confidentiality difficulties when parents known to practice. Ways of contacting patients other than by telephone when confidentiality a problem.

Decision: Patients to be told to contact surgery themselves for information and to consider advising private treatment where possible as considered easier to maintain privacy.

38. Pregnant epileptic: failed Microgynon

Patient aged 28 on Tegretol and Microgynon at own request. Other partners would have given same treatment and not considered this a problem. Patient happy to continue pregnancy but grounds for termination if requested.

Discussion: A check-list to look at when prescribing oral contraceptive. Update courses for family planning. Computer drug checks for females under 50.

Decision: To write protocol and design stamp for notes as checklist when prescribing oral contraceptive. To set up meeting on stamp design for various conditions.

39. Termination: medical reasons

Patient had previous normal pregnancy resulting in hydrocephalus and death of infant. Pregnant again but bleeding profusely. Referred. Seen weekly but no further communication with practice until a few months later when different partner written to about serious cardiac involvement. Referred tertiary centre where termination advised. No letter to practice about termination or where discharged to. Patient told about uterus abnormality for first time. Practice not told.

Discussion: Failure of communication between doctors. Still unknown why hospital involved second partner. Failure of hospital to advise practice by letter of termination and place patient discharged to. No follow-up arranged. Possible genetic counselling. Attitude of consultant and partners felt failure of communication was fault of hospital.

Decision: For partner involved to write to hospital about letters written to wrong doctor; no letters regarding termination; information regarding malformation of uterus; possible genetic counselling.

40. Fetal abnormality on ultrasound scan

Patient 18 weeks pregnant. Scan showed abnormality and partner advised by consultant to refer to main centre urgently. Patient telephoned by partner and asked to come to surgery for further information. Further telephone call from consultant to say not now considered to be important and further scan in 2 weeks was to be done.

Discussion: Unnecessary anxiety caused to patient by consultant's wrongly drawn conclusions before all facts available. General dissatisfaction with this particular consultant. Partner's handling of patient's questions over telephone and necessity of being circumspect to limit distress.

Decision: No decision.

41. Pregnant: no rubella immunity

Patient aged 38 with infertility problems. Had previous miscarriage but attempting pregnancy for 3–5 years. Screened for rubella with other tests. Laboratory denied receiving specimen. Repeat test requested over the telephone but not done. Patient subsequently became pregnant and had no cover.

Discussion: Partner congratulated on decision to do rubella check with infertility screening. Instructions in writing instead of over the telephone.

Decision: Check rubella status when screening for infertility. Be aware that immunity can become negative after a period of approximately 15 years.

42. Miscarriage at 20 weeks

Previous family history of antepartum haemorrhage at 20 weeks and spina bifida although no abnormality with this fetus.

Discussion: As above.

Decision: None.

43. and 44. Home delivery requests

Two friends, one primigravida and one para 1. Both patients appointed independent midwife having been told 'no' by partner to home delivery requests. Both referred to consultant for hospital delivery. Partner worried about patients at delivery and contract as may still be required to give antenatal care.

Discussion: Medical contract with patient. Whether antenatal but not obstetric care be given. Consultant's position and opinion regarding home delivery. Midwife's position.

Decision: Partner to discuss situation with consultant. Clarify contract in writing with FHSA and other protective body.

45. Oestradiol implant

Patient new to practice had been having implant privately. Told it could be done in surgery. Has since been arranged and completed.

Discussion: Procedure in surgery. Instruments required.

Decision: To enquire from drug company instruments required and costings.

46. Abnormal smear

Patient in her 20s reminded several times. Four years since last smear. Did eventually have smear and referred on abnormal result.

Discussion: Length of time between tests. Government guidelines of five years too long. Three years also felt to be too long.

Decision: To do tests every three years.

47. Abnormal smear

Patient invited to attend several times. Five years since last smear.

Discussion: As in number 46.

Decision: As in number 46.

48. Sudden death

Previous significant event—acute renal failure. Itinerant drug addict. Died in ambulance. ? accidental overdose.

Discussion: Nil.

Decision: Nil.

49. Sudden death

Male patient aged 70 with three-week history of back pain. Tests and x-rays normal. Treated as muscular. Later in severe pain. Seen at orthopaedic department, treated as acute orthopaedic problem and advised bed rest. Partner not convinced as patient too mobile and pain 'not right'. Patient collapsed 48 hours later with aortic aneurysm. Chest x-ray and pelvis x-ray normal prior to collapse. Femoral pulses not examined.

Discussion: Tests done in relation to diagnosis. Article in *British Medical Journal* on treating aortic aneurysm. Notifying specific doctor at hospital of diagnosis.

Decision: A reminder to be vigilant when patient presents with atypical back pain and no other relevant symptoms. To feel abdomens in men over 65 when opportunity presents (5 × more prevalent in men than women). Copy of *British Medical Journal* article to be circulated to all doctors.

50. Sudden death

Female patient died suddenly at home same day as husband died in hospital (registered elsewhere). Partner visited patient at home four days prior to death—no serious symptoms but looking after very ill husband at home. Confusion in practice following death. Relative already informed that possible coroner's case and postmortem but no information at reception with regard to death certificate. Police telephoned next day to say not notified.

Discussion: Communication system for reception staff to give necessary support to bereaved families. Confusion in public arena and no side room for distressed relatives. Notifying police (which had been done but not logged) and correct coroner for area. Death certificates.

Decision: Doctor will see bereaved families either in their own home or in surgery at appointed time and will inform them of procedure following death. Review system for issuing death certificates. Clarify with police which coroner is used and the non-registered call from practice.

51. Three sudden deaths

Three deaths all under 65 were discussed under one heading:
(a) Patient a major risk for vascular disease, ex-smoker, previous myocardial infarction, asthma—well controlled. Elevated blood pressure. Died myocardial infarction.
(b) Known malignancy, hospitalized for investigations. ? secondaries. Developed an irregular pulse and died suddenly—myocardial infarction.
(c) Subarachnoid haemorrhage. Heavy smoker who disregarded all advice—told nurse to mind her own business.

Discussion: As above.

Decision: Nil.

52. Sudden death

Patient collapsed and died despite being monitored for heart problems. Seen by surgeons and symptoms not severe enough to warrant surgery.

Discussion: As above.

Decision: Nil.

53. Sudden death

Baby with Down's syndrome died eight weeks after cardiac surgery. Results of postmortem showed superior vena cava blocked and thrombosed, vegetation on valves and bacterial endocarditis.

Discussion: Symptoms, and surprise at length of time child lived.

Decision: Nil.

54. Sudden death

Patient diagnosed hypertensive ten years earlier for which he received treatment. Three years later, he suffered a myocardial infarction and a further 2 years later left ventricular failure. He had been managed and monitored regularly over the years. All risk factors were taken into account and treated.

Discussion: As above.

Decision: Nil.

55. Sudden death

Patient had severe unstable asthma from childhood. On all possible medication and oral steroids plus nebulizer. He had been out on the previous day and was not particularly worse than on other occasions. He had an attack and died.

Discussion: As above.

Decision: Nil.

56. Sudden death. myocardial infarction

No previous history of heart disease. Previously treated for asthma but poor compliance with treatment. Seen three days before she died and advised to commence Becotide. Advised to stop smoking on previous occasions. Blood pressure when checked recently was 130/80. Cholesterol not checked as she was not considered to be in a risk category.

Discussion: As above.

Decision: All care given. No decision.

57. Sudden death due to left ventricular failure under 65

Patient was found dead in her flat. Had been hypertensive for twenty years. Intravenous pyelogram 15 years ago showed chronic pyelonephritis. Defaulted on follow-up appointments so disease not monitored regularly. Blood pressure control was not good but she was reluctant to increase treatment. Cholesterol levels were satisfactory. She smoked and had been given advice on this. Her electrolytes two years ago were normal. She had been seen twice recently by a physician for shortness of breath which was attributed to chronic bronchitis. There were no signs of heart failure. There was no record of alcohol intake in her notes.

Discussion: Regular monitoring of patient.

Decision: Patients suffering from hypertension to have their alcohol intake recorded.

58. Sudden death due to left ventricular failure under 65

Insulin dependent diabetic patient with multiple complications for which he was receiving treatment. Also receiving treatment for renal failure, left ventricular failure and retinopathy. He tended to do his own thing and ran his sugars high. Found dead in his car having died from acute left ventricular failure.

Discussion: As above.

Decision: Nil.

59. Sudden death, previous myocardial infarction: treated for elevated blood pressure

Died myocardial infarction. Previously treated for raised blood pressure. Well controlled on bendrofluazides. Lipids and electrolytes not done.

Discussion: As above.

Decision: ? patients on bendrofluazides to have electrolytes tested every three months.

60. Sudden death: peptic ulcer

Patient on cimetidine died from regurgitation of stomach contents. Postmortem revealed cardiorespiratory arrest. Peptic ulceration of oesophagus.

Discussion: Patient found dead. Had been well one hour previously. Previous history of gastric surgery and pyeloplasty. Heavy smoker with chronic cough. Seen two weeks previously asymptomatic.

Decision: Nothing to be done.

61. Sudden death

Previous history of hypertension. Treated two days previously for respiratory infection.

Discussion: Smoking habits not recorded, nor cholesterol levels. It was thought, however, that these were not indicated at the time. It was agreed that this patient was at risk and his smoking habits should have been recorded.

Decision: To record the smoking habits of all at-risk patients.

62. Sudden death: left ventricular failure

Patient treated both in hospital and in practice for left ventricular failure over the past 5/6 years. On medication and well controlled. No evidence of heart disease. Patient last attended complaining of respiratory infection. Treated and told to come back 2 weeks later. Came back—clear. Two days later came back with increased left ventricular failure. Sent for chest x-ray. Electrocardiogram showed no evidence of worsening failure.

Discussion: As above.

Decision: No decision.

63. Biliary disease and heart disease: sudden death

Patient found dead. A few days before his death he had called the doctor out twice and was treated for biliary pain.

Discussion: It was thought with hindsight that this may have been coronary rather than biliary pain. A discussion on the merits of cholesterol testing followed with reference to journals. The appointment system for scans at the local hospital was also discussed and it was pointed out that the appointment system there needed auditing.

Decision: No decision.

64. Sudden unexpected death: heart failure

Patient passed out at home. Doctor called out. Blood pressure 100/80. Called back later but patient had died. Reported to coroner. Postmortem revealed left ventricular failure, heart disease and carcinoma stomach.

Discussion: Question raised as to whether to put elderly patients who live alone into hospital. It was considered impossible to generalize as each case had to be treated on its own merit.

Decision: No decision.

65. Sudden death: ruptured heart

Patient collapsed. Past history of steroids, ruptured Achilles tendon, frail with thin skin. Not on oral steroids for some time but on inhaled steroids. Was better on this. Had oral and inhaled steroids stopped because there was no improvement to be seen at clinic, although patient felt better. Doctor was upset that medication had been stopped and phoned to say so. Patient seen for review, and agreed some objective improvement. Started on inhaled steroids again.

Discussion: Discussion followed over the use of steroids and anti-inflammatory preparations. Thought worth discussing the use of prophylactics and anti-inflammatory drugs. Also raised—advice to patients on calling out ambulances for severe chest pain. It was agreed that the quickest and safest measure for those suffering from severe chest pain was to dial 999.

Decision: To set up a discussion group on the use of prophylactic and anti-inflammatory drugs.

66. Myocardial infarction

Male patient aged 50 presented with history of two weeks of angina and severe symptoms for past 24 hours. Ambulance called and patient admitted. Had attended two well-man clinics. No hypertension shown on two recent blood pressure tests. No cholesterol test done before attack but slightly raised six weeks after.

Discussion: Family history discussed at clinic? Automatic cholesterol testing at clinic as some patients missed by following protocol. Protocol for admissions of myocardial infarction cases. Ambulance with defibrillator equipment coming for coronary calls.

Decision: Protocol for well-man clinic not to be changed with regard to cholesterol tests unless more similar cases present in the future. Always ask for ambulance with defibrillator in coronary cases and write to ask how often this occurs.

67. Myocardial infarction

Male patient aged 70, fit, recently retired. Sudden collapse. Had been vomiting for 24 hours when partner called. ? gastric flu. Admitted after resuscitation. Died 18 hours later. Hospital confused as to second sudden collapse.

Discussion: Diagnosis—atypical myocardial infarction. Postmortem results which showed dehydration.

Decision: No decision.

68. Myocardial infarction

47-year-old married man. Heavy smoker. Rejected invitations to well-man clinic. Seen rarely. Partner called 3 a.m. Patient complaining of tight chest pain radiating down left arm. Saw 45 minutes after symptoms started but pain present 3/4 days previously. Diagnosis: crescendo angina/small myocardial infarction. Admitted. Discharged after 3 days having had electrocardiogram etc. Tests normal. Concluded musculoskeletal and Brufen prescribed. Outpatient appointment 2 months. Seen again at home 3 days later with further chest pain. Collapsed at home one week later.

Discussion: Failure of health promotion scheme and inability to persuade patient to attend. Partner upset regarding failure of hospital to take diagnosis seriously. Felt stress test should have been performed before discharge and prophylaxis begun. Inappropriate outpatient appointment for 2 months in view of probable diagnosis and notification of non-attendance to clinic after death. Combined audit meeting with hospital staff regarding management of angina and contacting audit manager at hospital to ask if they would be interested.

Decision: To inform hospital consultant involved of outcome. To discuss management of angina at the next joint meeting of physicians and general practitioners.

69. Myocardial infarction—missed diagnosis

Patient with carcinomatosis deteriorating rapidly. Developed chest pains and gross oedema of lower legs. Increasing congestive heart failure. On MST and morphine. Left ventricular failure—admitted. Died 12 hours after admission.

Discussion: Infarct suspected three days previously but masked by MST. Treatment administered considered correct.

Decision: No decision.

70. Myocardial infarction: cardiac arrest

Male patient aged 50. No current illness. Slim. No apparent risk factors. Collapsed suddenly at home. Had complained of ache in shoulder two weeks previously but not severe. Autopsy confirmed large coronary thrombosis.

Discussion: Family history—none. Well-man clinic—had visited in last five years. Blood pressure normal. Defibrillator carried in doctor's car.

Decision: No decision.

71. Myocardial infarction

Male patient with classic chest pain. Heavy smoker but stopped five years ago. Not overweight. Very active until laminectomy. Long history of spinal problems. Blood pressure normal. Low renal threshold—glycosuria. Random blood sugar normal. Never had cholesterol check. No family history.

Discussion: As above.

Decision: No decision.

72. Undiagnosed myocardial infarction

59-year-old woman presented with upper respiratory infection, pleuritic chest pain, rapid pulse, pyrexial. Pericardial friction rub. Diagnosed angina. Refused to be admitted. Treated with antibiotics. Pain still there next day. Diagnosed pericarditis. Chest x-ray showed no abnormality. Blood tests taken and electrocardiogram. Changes apparent. ? undiagnosed myocardial infarction. Seen outpatients. ? viral pericarditis and myocarditis.

Discussion: Management when patient refuses to co-operate. An earlier electrocardiogram. Management during holiday periods for doctors.

Decision: Always do electrocardiogram within 24 hours when pericardial friction rub apparent. Find out why patient will not co-operate. Domiciliary visit.

73. Myocardial infarction: recovered: angina now

Six-month history of angina treated with glyceryl trinitrate and nifedipine. Patient stopped taking medication once the pain subsided and on being told her electrocardiogram was normal.

Discussion: Patient had been seen on other occasions for other reasons and could have been followed up. It was thought that she may have benefited from taking aspirin.

Decisions: (a) Patients with angina to be put on to aspirin as routine if suitable. This will be done opportunistically as patients are seen. (b) Partners to carry aspirin in bags at all times, half a tablet to be given if there is a suspected infarct.

74. Myocardial infarction: nothing of previous note

Recently registered with the practice. Usual new patient check-up, nothing of note. Electrocardiogram normal. Seen from time to time with pain in shoulder. Complained of retrosternal pain for two previous mornings. Thought to be suspicious and admitted. Diagnosis myocardial infarction. This patient was not thought to be at risk. His urine, blood pressure, cholesterol were all normal. Pain in shoulder not thought to be related to heart condition.

Discussion: As above.

Decision: Nothing to be done—all care given.

75. Discussion of one myocardial infarction (four on the list)

Presented with flu-like illness. Blood pressure 160/90. Went back to work. Seen as an emergency after fainting twice at work. He had been sick after the first faint. On examination, he looked ill, grey and sweating. Blood pressure 120/85. Cardiac enzymes suggested a coronary. Sent for urgent outpatient appointment. At clinic, blood pressure 171/110. Electrocardiogram normal. Diagnosis—simple faint. Raised creatine phosphokinase (CPK) attributed to falling.

Discussion: Issue raised for discussion about sending this patient back to work. Why did he faint and why did he vomit? The patient was not seen by a consultant at clinic. All the signs were that he had a coronary. One of the partners raised the point about a similar case where a simple illness was diagnosed after the same sort of symptoms. The patient now has severe heart disease. It was pointed out that it was of value to express concern to the consultant over the diagnosis, perhaps suggesting

an exercise test. Gut feelings are often confirmed. General practitioners do not question diagnoses enough.

Decision: Not to accept a hospital diagnosis if it goes against own judgement and to question the consultant concerned.

76. Pulmonary embolus

Female patient presented with pain and swelling of lower left leg. Indigestion. No examination done above knee. Admitted later with pulmonary embolus and patient said later that there was swelling up to groin.

Discussion: More comprehensive examination when patient presents with ankle swelling.

Decision: As above.

77. Pulmonary embolism after immobilization in plaster and taking oral contraceptives

Patient immobilized in plaster. Previous family history—father had suffered a deep vein thrombosis.

Discussion: As above.

Decision: Patients immobilized in plaster and taking oral contraceptives to be advised to stop taking them until mobile.

78. Pulmonary embolism many weeks after fracture

Developed an embolism many weeks after fracture. Now anticoagulated.

Discussion: As above.

Decision: Nil.

79. Deep vein thrombosis on oral contraceptive

Girl aged 14, first seen aged 12 with menorrhagia. History of 4 cycles of very heavy periods. Put on oral contraceptive with parental approval. Presented with 24-hour history of swollen left ankle up to mid-calf and tender lower calf muscles. Partner requested venogram but informed no longer done for deep vein thrombosis. Admitted. Diagnosis musculoskeletal. Bed rest. Swelling subsided. Taken off Pill. No confirmed diagnosis of deep vein thrombosis. Patient confused and frightened. Becoming neurotic. Partner worried for future treatment and contraception when needed and felt need to diagnose condition formally.

Discussion: Identification of deep vein thrombosis by clinical examination or venogram.

Decision: Venogram only positive way of identifying deep vein thrombosis. To re-refer patient on receiving discharge letter, possibly to gynaecologist. Enquiries to be made regarding diagnosis.

80. Cerebrovascular accident: discharged not on aspirin

Patient discharged following cerebrovascular accident not on aspirin. Subsequent trans ischaemic attack (TIA) and re-admitted. Discharged still not on aspirin.

Discussion: Merits of giving aspirin in such cases and results of various recent trials on such. Correct management of hypertension in elderly patients as a means of preventing strokes by possibly using more aggressive treatment.

Decision: To conduct audit on management of post-cerebrovascular events to be semi-retrospective and, in particular, to look at recent blood pressure checks. To conduct a second audit on postmyocardial infarct and angina patients.

81. Cerebrovascular accident: hypertension

Female patient aged 70 had hypertension for 30 years. Reasonably controlled over last four years.

Discussion: Acceptable blood pressure levels and risk of side effects if too vigorous treatment given. Protocol for ongoing treatment. Uniformity of treatment.

Decision: To give thought to protocol for ongoing treatment and discuss again at next practice meeting.

82. Cerebral haemorrhage

Male patient aged 62. In coma in hospital for three days. Very overweight. Diagnosed hypertensive at time of cerebrovascular accident. Blood pressure checked three months previously. Diastolic slightly raised. At previous practice, notes showed blood pressure raised but no diagnosis and no treatment. Now well controlled and losing weight.

Discussion: Detailed note search of new patients.

Decision: To write problems such as raised blood pressure across notes of new arrivals.

83. Stroke in a patient with diabetes

Admitted to hospital with a left-sided hemiparesis and a blood pressure of 230/210. Diagnosed as having pre-existing hypertension. On checking through records over the past two years, sugars and cholesterol levels normal. He was a non-smoker. His blood pressure readings over the past two years had fluctuated on two occasions, one 180/70 and another 160/100. His last seven readings averaged 153/82.

Discussion: It was difficult to decide whether he should have been treated as his blood pressure always returned to normal soon after it had been elevated. Treatment protocol for diabetics states treatment at 160/90 and lower if there are renal problems.

Decision: All care given. All tests carried out regularly and were within normal limits. Nothing else to be done.

84. Stroke in a 28-year-old

This young man suffered a stroke with no previous history. Resolved now and to stay on aspirin. Investigations do not indicate any other treatment. Blood pressure and cholesterol levels normal.

Discussion: As above.

Decision: Nothing to be done or could have been done to prevent this happening.

85. Left-sided hemiparesis: transient ischaemic attack

Previous history of hypertension and stroke. Diagnosed as having hypertension one year ago. Had a left-sided stroke eight years ago and also suffered from chronic obstructive airways disease. Recently suffered a deep vein thrombosis and was on anticoagulants for three months. When warfarin stopped, put back on aspirin. Two days later, he developed weakness in his left leg and diagnosed as having a TIA. There was no notification of anticoagulants being stopped at clinic. Blood pressure was normal. There were no carotid bruits.

Discussion: As above.

Decision: Nothing to be done.

86. Mild cerebrovascular accident

Previous history of hypertension treated with Adalat, heart disease treated with aspirin, TIA.

Discussion: The importance of physiotherapy starting as soon as possible after a stroke. There is no stroke service locally and, in order to get physiotherapy, patients have to be referred to a consultant if they are over 65. It was thought a protocol was needed, to be worked out with the consultant geriatricians, in order to manage strokes more effectively.

Decision: A letter to be written asking consultant geriatricians to discuss a protocol on stroke management.

87. Mild cerebrovascular accident

Recent 'over 75' health check. No problems. Blood pressure 150/100. Hypertensive for 4 years and on treatment. Six years ago had three episodes of dizziness, left carotid bruits, blurred vision and found to be suffering from raised cholesterol. Treated with aspirin, refused hospital treatment. Always attended for blood pressure check. Referred by nurse with right-sided facial weakness and elevated blood pressure. Diagnosed as having a mild cerebrovascular accident. Seen two weeks later with residual facial weakness. Blood pressure 140/80.

Discussion: As above.

Decision: To continue with aspirin and blood pressure control.

88. Left-sided cerebrovascular accident in a blind insulin dependent diabetic patient

Well controlled and well looked after. Last blood sugar 9.7. Making a good recovery.

Discussion: As above.

Decision: Nothing to be done.

89. Hypertension—250/150

Female patient aged 68 not seen by doctor for several years. Blood pressure reading of 250/150 discovered at new patient check. Partner saw patient who was angry and only came under duress. Did not admit. Investigated and treated with beta blockers. Blood pressure slow to respond. No other symptoms and no sign of any other related problems. Second line of treatment instigated and blood pressure now down to 180/100. Tight practice protocol for hypertension followed.

Discussion: Protocol—shown to be working well as to regular screenings for specific groups of patients. Results on computer and the possibility of having to trawl through notes for updating. A further terminal in the nurses' room in addition to the treatment room.

Decision: To record all blood pressure readings on computer. To consider a second terminal for nurses.

90. Diagnosis of diabetes

Female patient, heavy drinker. Liver biopsy—cirrhosis. Gastroscopy—pyloric lesions. Presented with vaginal discharge—treated. Complained four days later of polyuria and thirst. Glucose in urine. Given dietary advice and diastix. Not fully controlled and now on tablets.

Discussion: As above.

Decision: No decision.

91. Diagnosis of diabetes

Male patient aged 50. Lorry driver. Diabetes picked up at hypertension clinic. Blood sugar positive. Glycosuria. Seen at hospital. Diet sufficient. May continue to drive unless becomes insulin dependent.

Discussion: As above.

Decision: No decision.

92. Diagnosis of diabetes

Woman aged 32 presented with thirst. No family history of diabetes. Three pregnancies with no evidence of diabetes. Seen in outpatients and treatment resolved.

Discussion: Failure of communication. Future care and treatment.

Decision: Patient should continue to be seen at hospital clinic. To continue present drug regime.

93. Newly diagnosed insulin dependent diabetic patient

Presented with a five-day history of weight loss, thirst and nausea. Admitted to hospital, rehydrated, started on insulin and is doing well. Previous history: wheezy bronchitis one year ago. Seen three times in five years, no steroids. Seen at follow-up. No problems.

Discussion: As above.

Decision: No decision.

94. Diabetes: poor vision

Single male patient in late seventies lost sight in one eye. Late onset diabetic. Referred diabetic screening clinic but not been since and denies receiving appointments. Attended surgery clinic 2 years ago for full check but otherwise only attends for other complaints. Control good—no tablets needed. Bilateral early cataracts. Referred optician—visual acuity dropped. Now severely disabled. Referred urgently to ophthalmic surgeon. Not seen for 3 months. Bilateral glaucoma and virtually blind. Says will commit suicide if loses sight completely.

Discussion: Consistent delay in cases being seen (approximately 6 weeks) by ophthalmic department and feeling let down. Patient poor complier and doubt about putting drops in eyes. Could have received clinic invitations but not understood. Protocol for referrals of glaucoma and possible future direct referrals by opticians. Clarification of protocol for emergency referrals. Hospital mechanism for informing practice regarding non-attendance at clinics and outpatient appointment system. Subject for possible future audit.

Decision: To write to secretary of department to enquire if appointments for clinic sent. To write to audit officer at hospital to enquire if a joint project could be undertaken and investigate possible funding.

95. Diabetic ketoacidosis

15-year-old boy presented with vomiting, headache. Blood sugar 20. No ketones in urine. Repeat blood sugar 28 after two hours. Admitted. Discharged but not followed up as under diabetic care elsewhere. Further episode when partner saw at home, blood sugar 34.8. Reduced blood sugar to 20 and tried to keep patient at home but mother suffers regular crises of confidence and telephoned diabetic liaison nurse who advised to admit.

Discussion: Difficulty of treating and educating patient with liaison nurse countermanding instructions without consultation. Family conditions not conducive to keeping sugar levels down. Patient not keeping to diet. Treatment at hospital—family not happy. Accuracy of BM stix. Need to educate relatives in importance of regular tests and keeping of records. Less care offered than normal because under hospital care and the possibility of a diabetic clinic at practice improving

standards at home and give more confidence to patients. Possibility of liaison nurse attending such a clinic. Role of practice nurses.

Decision: To take over control if possible. Partner to ask hospital to see only once a year to let practice reinforce role. Partner to communicate with diabetic liaison nurse.

96. Diabetic: sixth nerve palsy

Male patient aged 73 presented with double vision right eye. No other symptoms. Diagnosed palsy and referred. Urine test at hospital positive for glucose. Patient hypertensive and attends practice for blood pressure checks. Last urine test for glucose at practice four years ago—negative. Mild diabetic—diet alone.

Discussion: Merits of referral to ophthalmologist as against neurologist. Urine tests in well-man clinic.

Decision: To do annual urine tests for glucose in neuropathy patients.

97. Hypoglycaemia

Patient on insulin—poorly controlled. Presented with hypoglycaemia symptoms which had been present throughout previous night. Said tests done but thought BM stix faulty because not registering. Partner concerned that other patients may not know correct usage. Patient had no glucagon.

Discussion: Education of patients and their partners with regard to testing and handling of hypoglycaemic attacks by direct questioning. Necessity of availability of glucagon and other quick-acting treatments. Shelf life of glucagon (approximately 2 years).

Decision: Computer search of all insulin patients—glucagon. Check patients' supplies of glucagon up to date. Each patient to have necessary kit. Education of patients and their partners on injection technique and recognition of imminent hypoglycaemic attack.

98. Amputation of toe: insulin dependent diabetic patient

Patient in early fifties does not conform to dietary advice or treatment regime. This patient is seen privately by a retired physician who supervises his treatment. He was persuaded to attend NHS clinics but fell out with the consultant. Described as 'a law unto himself', he does not conform to his treatment plan despite the efforts of clinic staff.

Discussion: Preventable outcome but impossible to force a patient to accept treatment.

Decision: No decision.

99. Amputation of toe: non-insulin dependent diabetic patient

Patient with microvascular complications, retinopathy and obesity. Blood sugar and fructosamine not under control. Had one toe amputated.

Discussion: The merits of different approaches to patients who will not comply with treatment. It was acknowledged that patients have to be responsible for themselves and their motivation for change. It was thought to be a good idea to identify all the poor compliers and discuss a strategy for educating them and persuading them to comply with treatment, possibly in conjunction with the diabetic liaison nurse.

Decisions: (a) Identify all poor diabetic treatment compliers. (b) Put these on agenda for next practice meeting. (c) Discuss a strategy for education and persuasion possibly in conjunction with diabetic liaison nurse.

100. Amputation: insulin dependent diabetic patient

64-year-old for partial amputation of right foot. This patient has a multitude of problems: he is partially sighted, has vascular disease and has already had his left foot partially amputated. He now has severe problems with his right foot which is infected and difficult to manage. The hospital has tried to sort this problem out to no avail. It is not a problem of incorrect treatment and the decision to amputate rests with the surgeons.

Discussion: As above.

Decision: Well managed, no decision.

101. Lost macula function: insulin dependent diabetic patient

Patient was being looked after by the eye hospital and had previously had laser treatment which had held the blindness back for some time. He was being monitored at the local hospital diabetic clinic where his sugars ran between 9 and 12 and were improving. His last HbA1 was raised. He attended his reviews regularly although he did not monitor his own blood sugars.

Discussion: A discussion followed about the relationship between diabetic control and complications with reference to literature concerned.

Decision: No decision.

102. Diabetic: cut finger

Patient severe diabetic but very unconcerned regarding diet, etc. Well controlled. Waited four days before presenting because already had appointment. Needed stitching. Healed well. No problems.

Discussion: Regular diabetic checks confirm system working well.

Decision: No decision.

103. Diabetic amputation

Insulin dependent late onset diabetic. Previously took himself off tablets and never bothered with diet. Black area developed on foot and subsequent amputation. Treated by hospital since then. Never comes to practice.

Discussion: As above.

Decision: No decision.

104. Diabetic: poor control

Patient aged 75 on diet and tablets. Mentally subnormal. Blood sugars taken by son show very poor control. Had one cataract but otherwise no other side-effects. Cuts and bruises heal well.

Discussion: Further intervention needed?

Decision: No further medical intervention needed at this time.

105. Blood sugar—88

Male patient aged 80 seen frequently in practice. Lives alone. Partner called by home help. Wobbly, slight temperature, urine frequency. ? urinary tract infection. Drugs started. Returned later to re-assess, anticipating possible night call and tested for sugar—88. Admitted.

Discussion: Rapid onset of diabetes. Long list of ailments and drugs. Had recent over-75 check. No abnormality. Value of over-75 checks and any prior avoidance action that could have been taken.

Decision: Nothing more could have been done in addition to the regular medical checks received and the partner was congratulated by his colleagues on the thoroughness of his assessment.

106. Unstable diabetes in a 15-year-old

Patient became ill and unstable but refused admission to hospital. Monitored at home every two hours and his insulin adjusted accordingly. He was unable to do his paper round so his mother did it for him. Unfortunately, while she was delivering papers a 'flasher' jumped out and she dropped all of the papers in the canal and ran home. Her son was so amused he couldn't stop laughing which brought his blood sugars back to normal.

Discussion: One of the partners also pointed out that there was a diagnostic lesson to be learned from the treatment of this child. Prior to diagnosis he became enuretic, which was attributed to break down of his parents' marriage. Later, he was brought in to surgery in a moribund state and found to have diabetes.

Decision: Examine all children presenting with enuresis for diabetes.

107. Epileptic fit after 9 years

Male patient aged 41 had been on anticonvulsants for ten years. Had three grand mal convulsions. Last seen at hospital seven years ago. Partner satisfied with blood levels and decided to reduce dosage with a view to taking patient off drug completely if successful. No fits until patient went on recent holiday and forgot to take drugs for four days. Now lost driving licence and back on full dosage.

Discussion: Partner's responsibility with regard to driving. Had not previously given up driving and partner now felt responsible by reducing drugs. Confidentiality aspect. Value of routine blood levels even if asymptomatic. Possible annual review.

Decision: To take care before reducing dosage or changing drug. To review past medical history very carefully before making a decision.

108. Epileptic fit

Schoolboy had fit at school. Staff unaware of previous fit and diagnosis as mother unwilling to tell anyone. Discharged from hospital on slow release Tegretol after initial diagnosis but changed to ordinary Tegretol. Now back on slow release Tegretol.

Discussion: Advantages of slow release Tegretol—more even dosage throughout day. Possible change of all epileptic patients to slow release Tegretol. Paediatric discharges and dangers of diagnosis not being revealed.

Decision: Only to change patients with control problems to slow release Tegretol.

109. Right-sided hemiparesis with grand mal

Past history of myocardial infarction ten years before. Exercise electrocardiogram normal. The following year, a second myocardial infarction. One year ago, lipids 6.9. Cholesterol 1.5. Seen urgently with right-sided hemiparesis. No power right side, dysphagia. Discharged 4 weeks later but readmitted a further 4 weeks later with a grand mal convulsion. Put on to anticonvulsants. CT scan revealed left-sided infarct. Shortly after had another fit, medication increased to 300 mg. Discharged 2 months later from day hospital. Is ataxic, but some power back. Asked to prescribe Prozac for depression but reluctant to do so as this may cause further fits. Prognosis poor.

Discussion: As above.

Decision: No decision.

110. Epileptic taken off medication against wishes: had a fit

This 82-year-old patient, diagnosed as suffering from epilepsy 10 years ago and having had his last fit seven years ago, came to the clinic for a repeat prescription. It was decided to check his phenobarbitone and phenytoin level, which were subsequently found to be subclinical. It was thought he possibly did not now require medication and was referred to the geriatricians for confirmation. He was subsequently seen and it was agreed to withdraw medication. Patient displeased and subsequently had a large fit. He is now back on anticonvulsants.

Discussion: A discussion followed concerning the difficulties with subclinical levels. Reference was made to a paper in the *British Medical Journal* about the timing of taking levels and how this affects outcome.

Decision: Listen to what the patient has to say and do not rely on blood levels.

111. Epileptic fit: seen at home

Fits from childhood. Called out and diazepam given. Now trying to get epilepsy under control.

Discussion: As above.

Decision: To get fits under control.

112. Multiple sclerosis/brain tumour

Confirmed multiple sclerosis. Now unable to walk. Lengthy period of time before diagnosis confirmed. Matter discussed with patient before diagnosis. Requires support and discussion.

Discussion: Forward look at support system in rural community for chronic illness. Support system available to another known multiple sclerosis patient.

Decision: To hold clinical meeting to discuss resources available to patients with chronic illness with health visitor and nurses present.

113. Asthma: urgent admission

Patient girl aged 2. Mother picked up child from childminder. Wheezing a little. Telephoned partner who told mother to bring child to surgery for check. Child sweating profusely and ill. Very quiet chest. Mother asthmatic but did not recognize symptoms. Child had only one previous mild wheezing attack. Nebulized and admitted.

Discussion: Partner's immediate response following non-urgent telephone call. Mother's guilt at leaving child with minder and not recognizing symptoms. Significance of very quiet chest—no air entry.

Decision: Always to see young children if wheezing present.

114. Asthma: urgent visit

The need for a uniform policy on steroid therapy. Huge variations at present in methodology. Would be helpful for brittle asthmatics if all doctors treated patients in same way.

Discussion: Dosage, especially in children.

Decision: To discuss future meeting.

115. Asthmatic patient: refused appointment

Difficult father who can cause trouble. Patient has been in adolescent unit. Asked for appointment when fully booked Friday afternoon. Told to telephone Saturday if worse for emergency Saturday appointment. Patient did not return until Monday when considerably worse and required urgent treatment. Patient advised correctly.

Discussion: New appointment system which is working well.

Decision: No decision.

116. Asthma

Four cases of acute exacerbation of asthma discussed under one heading. All of these patients were known to the practice. They attended surgery regularly and were on regular therapy.

Discussion: It was pointed out that all of these cases may be attributed to failure of therapy. Nothing else to be done.

Decision: No decision.

117. Hospital admission for asthma

Child known to practice and attended clinic regularly. Prone to instability at times. She was not big enough to take prophylactics regularly and as such her asthma medication became insufficient at this time.

Discussion: Prophylactic treatment for asthma.

Decision: No decision.

118. Severe asthma patient in extremis

Had to be resuscitated in hospital after severe asthma attack.

Discussion: Preventive treatment, Ventolin and peak flow monitoring.

Decision: Nothing to be done.

119. Hospital admission for asthma

Admitted to hospital after a 999 call. Seen the day before, cough and purulent sputum. All medication increased and told he would be seen next day. Family rang 999 and admitted to hospital. Now seen regularly and asthma under control.

Discussion: As above.

Decision: Nothing to be done.

120. Acute asthma overnight stay in hospital

Registered two years ago but did not give a history of asthma. Smokes 20 per day. Presented with a heavy cold and wheezy chest, peak flow 350. Treated with Ventolin and told to come back for review but did not keep appointment. Five months later, she called doctor and was admitted. Put on nebulizer, inhalers and reducing steroids. Next day her peak flow was normal when seen by one of the partners. At this visit she was referred to the asthma clinic but failed to keep her appointment. Described as very disorganized, this patient has called out the doctor on subsequent occasions to treat her asthma.

Discussion: As above.

Decision: All newly diagnosed patients to be referred to asthma clinic in order to receive better education about their condition.

121. Acute asthma

Sore throat treated with erythromycin. Three days later back with chronic hacking cough, throat improved, chest wheezy, peak flow 250, using Ventolin occasionally. Started on a course of steroids 30 mg per day and a Bricanyl inhaler. Six days later still bad cough, peak flow improved at 350. Generally unwell. Mother in panic state—not satisfied. Saw consultant two weeks later, who suggested Pulmicort and a peak flow meter. On an inhaler for some time, although there was nothing on the front sheet of her records to indicate that she had asthma and no record of repeat prescriptions.

Discussion: Possibility that this attack had a psychological component to it with the death of her grandfather.

Decision: No decision.

122. Acute asthma emergency visit

Three-week history of pain and bronchospasm. Out of steroids. Seen with chest wall pain? start of shingles. One week later chest infection treated with antibiotics and reducing steroids. One month later, acute asthma treated with steroids and Becloforte. Brufen stopped until off steroids. Seen by consultant two weeks later for chronic cardiac failure, chronic airways disease and arthritis. Report states expiratory wheeze nothing marked.

Discussion: As above.

Decision: Encourage asthma patients to stay with one doctor.

123. Hospital admission for asthma

First diagnosed when treated for a wheezy cough with Ventolin and antibiotics. Seen six months later with a mild asthma attack. Ventolin prescribed. Repeat prescriptions given twice during year. Over the past twelve months, seen as an emergency on five occasions. Treated with Ventolin and antibiotics on the fifth occasion. Treatment altered to include Becotide. Three months later put on soluble prednisolone as well as Ventolin and Becotide but was transferred from inhalers to volumatic. On a routine visit to hospital the child's mother was told he did not have asthma despite the condition being diagnosed two years previously. Admitted when the child developed an acute asthma attack and became extremely poorly. Mother unaware how ill child was. Discharged next day and seen by partner. Mother will not accept diagnosis. Does not like the idea of her child being asthmatic.

Discussion: As above.

Decision: Set up a protocol for diagnosing and treating asthma with a view to setting up an asthma clinic.

124. Hospital admission for asthma

Presented with breathlessness and dry cough. Chest clear. Peak flow 450. Treated with Ventolin and told to come for follow up. Eleven days later, referred herself to casualty and admitted. Peak flow 180. Patient fainted and thought to have hyperventilated. Nebulized. Peak flow 440—discharged. Treated later by general practitioner with Becotide, Ventolin and given a peak flow meter. History: known asthmatic, had stopped taking Intal. Previous episode of hyperventilation. Not seen with chest problems since then, until this episode.

Discussion: Asthma management and need to give advice at follow-up.

Decision: No decision.

125. Asthma attack, nebulizer missing

Partner on call received call from patient who had just arrived from Malta and was having a severe asthma attack. Doctor stopped at surgery to pick up one of the two nebulizers available to the practice. No nebulizer available and wasted precious time searching. Patient was very ill and a potential fatality. Ambulance called on 999 with nebulizer on board. Patient was admitted to hospital. Nebulizer found in the back of partner's car and the other nebulizer was on loan and had not been returned.

Discussion: As above.

Decisions: (a) One nebulizer always to be kept in a known place in nurses' room. If taken out by doctor on call to be replaced next morning. (b) Any nebulizer loaned out to be returned in one day.

126. Non-accidental injury

Patient one of four children. Father noticed bruising caused by a slap after the child had spilled tea. He reported this to the doctor. Mother admitted to causing the injury which was slight, and the child had gone to live with her grandmother. Social services involvement with this family has been good, as has support from all other agencies including child psychiatry. Mother did not always attend case conferences or attend follow-up. She also complained of being depressed, although this was thought to be reactive. All that could be done was, and was well supported from all agencies.

Discussion: As above.

Decision: No decision.

127. Congenital dislocation of hip

Child with congenital dislocation of hip picked up at birth and kept under observation. At six weeks her condition was thought to be stable by both general practitioner and paediatrician. At six months an x-ray revealed a truly displastic hip. This condition was not missed. At follow-up the child appeared satisfactory. There were no delays in picking up the condition.

Discussion: As above.

Decision: No decision.

128. Undescended testicle

Child admitted for appendicectomy and diagnosed as undescended testicle. Notes read "both testes have descended".

Discussion: Testicles should be brought down before the age of three but, unfortunately, for this child it was thought his testicle was descended.

Decision: Nil.

129. Acute renal failure

Male patient aged 31. Heroin addict. Temporary resident. Moves around a great deal. Presented with chest infection and dental problems. Had methadone from previous doctor. Reappeared clear of drugs and needing treatment for dental problems. Returned with severe pain in arm and wanted drugs. Given non-steroidals. Temporary residence certificate lapsed. Was asked to re-register but did not. Is known to have registered with another practice who rang for information on case.

Discussion: Notes of temporary residents. Should they be sent back and photocopies kept? Circulation of information for temporary residents to other general practitioners particularly concerning drug addicts.

Decision: To notify FHSA of particular cases where patient is moving around, in particular when trying to obtain drugs. To check computer which shows three-month residency but not that it had lapsed. Notes should be sent back to own general practitioner but photocopies kept. Memo to be sent round everyone in practice about such patients for information.

130. Eye trauma

Female patient with acutely sore eye. Examined by partner and sent to hospital for further examination. Dilated pupil which eased spasm and reduced pain.

Discussion: As above.

Decision: Reminder that in cases of acute eye pain, dilation of pupils reduces spasm and pain.

131. Suicide

Patient was 36-year-old man living alone. He had worked at his job from leaving school and had recently been made redundant. There was no previous history of depression. Postmortem revealed that he had hacked himself to death.

Discussion: As above.

Decision: No decision.

132. Suicide attempt/brain tumour

Male patient, mid-20s, came to practice after brain tumour diagnosed. Feeling amongst the doctors not enough being done to keep in contact with the case, with general absence of letters and reports from regional centre with regard to tumour. Letter written to neurosurgeon at regional centre asking for information. Patient now in permanent psychiatric care.

Discussion: Role of general practitioner when regional centre involved and whether general practitioner should see patient first before each visit, even in an emergency, in order to keep updated. Policy for admissions and discharges: notes to be pulled at intervals to keep in contact; list of incidences to be made to see when visits might be appropriate; telephone review.

Decision: To enquire more closely and regularly from family and regional centre, when involved, and to raise general level of awareness. More emotional support to be given. Discharge slips and patient's notes to be put on doctors' desks for decision to visit or phone. The duty doctor to deal with this if usual doctor away.

133. Attempted suicide

Very emaciated female patient aged 75. Had asthma/chronic obstructed airways disease/osteoporosis for long time. Very anaemic and in great pain. Took overdose of sleeping pills, possibly with husband's knowledge but not help. Recovered.

Discussion: Merits of giving service by prolonging life when patient in real distress and when to withdraw.

Decision: No decision.

134. Three cases of overdose

Three cases subsumed under one heading. Patient number one took an overdose of paracetamol. This may have been a reaction to domestic circumstances. She had not shown any psychological problems previously. Patients number two and three were both well known to the practice. They have been monitored by both the practice and all other available agencies.

Discussion: All support that could be given was provided. None of these instances involved a really serious attempt at suicide, although they were viewed as cries for help.

Decision: Nil.

135. Overdose

Patient had not attended the practice for some years. There was no warning of the impending event. Probably occurred as a result of problems with a broken relationship.

Discussion: The event was unpredictable and unpreventable.

Decision: No decision.

136. Overdose of paracetamol

Young woman took overdose of paracetamol. Patient suffering from hormone problem coupled with social and personal problems.

Discussion: This was described as a tragedy waiting to happen. Counselling and psychological support offered but not taken up. Felt that somehow they had let this patient down but had offered all they could. Nothing else to be done.

Decision: No decision.

137. Overdose of drink and drugs

Patient overdosed despite being under regular medical supervision. Patient a law unto himself who went on binges every so often.

Discussion: Nothing to be done.

Decision: No decision.

138. Overdose of Prothiaden

New patient with a previous history of mental instability took overdose of Prothiaden.

Discussion: Difficulty felt on making a decision about this patient. He was seen by a locum and discussion centred around possibly producing a protocol so that locums are aware of prescribing practices of the group.

Decision: No decision.

139. Overdose of drugs and alcohol

Patient well known to the practice and taken an overdose on previous occasion. Offered help from all agencies but refuses to accept it.

Discussion: Nothing to be done.

Decision: No decision.

140. Assault

Family unit of two parents, one son aged 2 and one daughter aged 1. Father has two jobs, low income and will not apply for income support. Children frequently ill with minor complaints and many unnecessary house calls asked for. Wife assaulted but no evidence of physical abuse of children. Problems caused by social circumstances.

Discussion: Increased demands on practice for trivial complaints very often at unsocial hours, possibly to avoid seeing the same doctor. General concern for family. Health visitor has visited frequently to try to build up relationship, confidence and possible opening up on the marital situation. Possibility of referring family to the social services for help.

Decision: To ask health visitor to put pressure on father to apply for social aid by filling in appropriate forms.

141. Died in fire

Child died from smoke inhalation. Partner at scene. Mother rescued and attempts made by practice to contact help agency (CRUSE). Now moved out of area.

Discussion: As above.

Decision: No decision.

142. Chlamydia urethritis

Patient counselled for vasectomy but delayed because of dysuria intermittent for 15 years. Noticed discharge and pain for a few days every 3/4 years. Swabs positive. Prescribed tetracycline. Repeat chlamydial swab positive. Wife not treated but matter discussed. ? re-infection or drug therapy not effective.

Discussion: Whether to treat at practice or refer. Confidentiality aspect of results of tests.

Decision: To refer all patients with urethral discharges for appropriate investigations at hospital.

143. Measles

Boy aged $2\frac{1}{2}$ vaccinated 15 months ago, presented with snuffly type illness and rash but otherwise well. No contact history.

Discussion: Very mild symptoms possibly due to vaccination. Unusual disease nowadays but notifiable.

Decision: To be alert for possibility of measles in children even after vaccination.

144. Pyosalpinx

Patient aged 47 with coil *in situ* presented with vaginal discharge and heavy periods. Coil removed and smear taken. Coil checked two years previously. Swab taken from discharge—*E Coli*. Treated with trimethoprim. Presented again two months later with flu-like symptoms, further discharge and crepitations in lungs. Treated with amoxycillin. Seen two weeks later with lower abdominal pain, lump left side, bleeding vaginally for three weeks. Tiredness. Bloods taken. White cell count 14 200. Rigors. Referred. Pelvis full of pus. Salpingectomy performed.

Discussion: Use of coils and unusual infection in stable relationship. Length of flu-like symptoms and possibility of antibiotic treatment masking other symptoms. Future treatment of vaginal discharges and infections.

Decision: To check patients with coil annually. Caution if flu-like illness continuing and to think more broadly as to other causes.

145. Excision of infected toenails

Nurses asked if this procedure could be undertaken in surgery as removal at hospital with wedges often resulted in infection.

Discussion: As above.

Decision: Partner said he was happy to undertake this procedure in surgery.

146. Legionnaire's disease

Male patient aged 51 presented with viral illness. Sweats, confusion but very little to hear in chest. Not been abroad or had contact with Legionnaire's disease. ? contracted through air conditioning system at factory where he worked. No other people suffering similar symptoms but could have been put down to flu and not reported.

Discussion: Ways of picking up and recording relevant flu-like symptoms among vulnerable patients. Recording—practice does record occupation but not where patients work. Possibility of telephoning place of work if worried and do search.

Decision: To bear in mind possibility of Legionnaire's disease when patients present with flu-like symptoms but no practical course of action felt to be of use at present time.

147. Probable HIV positive

Partner felt that the patient was likely to be HIV positive, although patient had refused test. Situation dealt with by trainee who persuaded patient to have test. Seen by consultant but felt to have been prevaricating.

Discussion: Safety measures for staff when treating HIV patients, such as blood taking and possible needle stick injury. Hospital policy on needle stick injury available but complicated. Information given to meeting from practice known to be well used to dealing with such patients. Necessity of diagnosis being known to whole team and to treat as any other patient.

Decision: Diagnosis to be known to whole team. To treat as positive if suspected but unconfirmed. A further meeting planned with nurses to discuss protocol. A practice policy to be initiated following meeting.

148. Malaria

Temporary resident. Seen by another general practitioner on return from Kenya. Developed fevers. Bloods taken. Diagnosis made and treatment started. Came to stay with parents. Very ill. Falciparum malaria diagnosed. Admitted, discharged and re-admitted psychotic. Family history: mother manic depressive. Partner concerned about wrong initial diagnosis and treatment which could have resulted in patient's death.

Discussion: Patient's illness and possibility of precipitating psychosis. Diagnosis and management of different types of malaria. Treatment with chloroquine.

Decision: Partner to telephone Hospital for Tropical Diseases for advice on management. To decide on practice policy for treatment of malaria.

149. Tuberculosis of the bladder

Patient presented with haematuria and admitted to a two-year history of urine infections. No previous history on records. Had not told doctors about his urinary symptoms. A previously raised erythrocyte sedimentation rate (ESR) settled after treatment. No complaints of night sweats.

Discussion: This was a chance finding. The patient did not have anything wrong with urine two years previously, neither had anything abnormal shown when he attended outpatients with a different problem.

Decision: No decision.

150. Tuberculosis meningitis: bizarre presentation

Child first diagnosed as having viral infection with nothing specific found. Seen again two days later, unwell, temperature up and down, sore throat, sick, right cervical node. Midstream urine test to exclude urinary tract infection. To come back for blood tests, ESR, monospot, full blood count. Results of blood test did not fit viral picture: ESR 52, white cell count 18 000. Spoke to paediatrician who thought it may be glandular fever. Two days later test came back negative. Nothing else to find except added sounds at left base. Mother said that the child had been bitten when at the park. Blood sent to public health laboratory. Seen by paediatrician two days later and admitted—

nothing specific. Two days later being sick. ? raised intracranial pressure. Lumbar puncture to look for meningitis. Given intravenous antibiotics. Diagnosed as having tuberculous meningitis, receiving steroids, getting better. No positive culture to date (takes six weeks).

Discussion: As above.

Decision: Keep monitoring children who are non-specific.

151. Meningitis

Temporary resident aged 14. Mother thought he had chickenpox. Relevant advice given over the telephone from protocol but recommended to speak to doctor. Parents rang later to report temperature, aches and sickness. Itchy blisters. Telephoned again $2\frac{1}{2}$ hours later—much worse and difficult to rouse. Partner diagnosed meningococcal meningitis and admitted. Partner unable to administer penicillin as patient allergic and asthmatic. Rang hospital to have alternative treatment ready. Recovered.

Discussion: Faster diagnosis. Staff acted correctly on information given over the telephone. Parents not originally concerned resulting in poor communication. See every reported rash. Carry something other than penicillin— ? chloramphenicol.

Decision: To rely on fast ambulance rather than carry chloramphenicol as an alternative to penicillin.

152. Meningitis

Patient diagnosed meningococcal meningitis. Penicillin administered.

Discussion: As above.

Decision: Always to remember to carry penicillin and administer intravenously, if possible.

153. Family antagonism about treatment

Elderly male patient aged 81 reasonably fit until gastric disturbance. Admitted. Hypertension found during investigations. Blood pressure extremely high. Consultant advised beta blocker drug and partner prescribed following lengthy discussion with patient concerning possible side-effects. Advice regarding danger of stroke also given. Saw one month later and drugs received but not taken on advice of relatives. Blood pressure too high to record. Patient started to take drug. Became ill with septicaemia and admitted. Relatives very angry and accused partner of poisoning patient. Difficult telephone conversation.

Discussion: Partner felt called to account. Potential litigation case. Aggressive relatives and possibility of fabricating evidence whilst under stress. Care taken to explain drug and follow-up by practice. Nurses approached requesting information, as they often are for clarification. Awkward situations and the need to keep staff informed. Possible medico-legal flag system needed.

Decision: To be always aware of medico-legal problems when dealing with difficult patients and relatives. To explain everything fully and keep strictly to the rules. To bring up any potentially difficult situations at the monthly meeting for staff to keep everyone informed. Flag system for notes.

154. Chronic leg ulcers: unco-operative patient

Female patient aged 72. Suffered from leg ulcers for many years. District nurses report that every time ulcer is partially healed, patient evades treatment. Present ulcer for approximately 14 months. Referred to dermatologist. Suggested treatment carried out but after few weeks patient wanted change. Very difficult and negative patient. Possible psychological problems.

Discussion: Drug regime. General health of patient and tests done. Hygiene in nurses' treatment room. Treatment of long-standing ulcers by dermatologist in Leeds.

Decision: Change of drug regime. Change of localized therapy as tried in Leeds. To continue with practice as patient wishes despite now living elsewhere. Psychological support to continue to be given.

154. Further discussion of above patient and failure to accept medical advice

Patient now living out of immediate area. Demands frequent change of treatment. Insistence on unsuitable treatments.

Discussion: Justification to advise to change doctor in view of total unco-operation. Expenses involved of frequent new bandages, etc. District nurse handling of issue.

Decision: For senior partner to see patient when she next attends. For swab to be taken at next visit. For district nurse to discuss handling of such cases with manager at next meeting.

155. Unnecessary screening of the elderly

Patient seen at home previously by nurse and in practice by partner when tests completed but not noted on computer. Patient received letter for screening and despite being very frail, attended surgery on her own. Nurse worried about patient's health, wasting patient's time and appointment time. Communication breakdown of this type has happened on previous occasions.

Discussion: Procedures for notifying secretaries of screenings done and entering details on computer. Completing stickers in notes and dated letter questionnaires for filing in letter section of notes.

Decision: To notify secretaries of all screenings done by doctors when patient attends ordinary surgery. To tell patient what screening has been done to avoid unnecessary future visits.

156. Therapeutic referrals and difficult consultations

Three therapeutic referrals of 'heart-sink' patients and one taken off list. Allocated new doctor visited patient and insisted she behave or he would not keep her. Patients with personality problems and constant complaining. Dislike of referral course of action for this reason.

Discussion: Necessity of referrals sometimes to placate patient. Patient removed from list and subsequent problem with phone calls requesting to come back.

Decision: A possible topic for future audit.

157. Fractured elbow

Female patient aged 65 on steroids walked in to see nurse having fallen and shattered elbow. In considerable pain with five breaks. Partner called and ambulance control called for ambulance within 20 minutes. Ambulance control difficult with receptionist and said $1\frac{1}{2}$ hours wait and would send car. Partner called and requested 'blue light'. Ambulance crew surly. Nurses felt authority being challenged.

Discussion: Different degrees of what constitutes emergency and need for caution in requesting 'blue light' so as not to devalue. Future procedure for calling ambulances. Action needed regarding this particular case.

Decision: No further action required in this instance. If possible, doctors should ring for ambulances in future. Considered to be more straightforward and cause less difficulty. Person calling for ambulance should always state acceptable time lapse according to emergency.

158. Section 2

Patient sexually abused as child. Very disturbed and developed schizophrenic-type illness. Now married with two children. Very aggressive and threatening. Admitted twice under section 2. Stopped taking medication but now on Depixol administered by community psychiatric nurse every two weeks.

Discussion: Patient stopping taking medication and the possibility of giving injections before due while patient still amenable. Sections generally and the use of section 4 (72 hours). Role of social workers.

Decision: Out-of-hours telephone numbers for duty social worker given. To be more aware of section 4 and use only in absolute emergency.

159. No psychiatric advice available

Patient in need of urgent psychiatric advice. Depressed and ? sectionable. Partner did not feel he could section with social worker as patient compulsive liar. Local hospital did not know who was 'on call'. Eventually found psychiatrist but at a distance and unwilling to visit that day.

Discussion: Chaotic psychiatric cover at hospital in question. Time wasted by partner in trying to make necessary arrangements.

Decision: For partner to write to psychiatrist with responsibility for area regarding on-call cover and contact for acute psychiatric opinion. To discuss matter with community psychiatric nurse.

160. Private referral for back pain

Patient complaining severe back pain referred privately by partner. Patient sent bill for £50. Husband unemployed, financially unstable and refused to pay. Said at no time had he agreed to his wife having private treatment and said practice should pay as they were at fault.

Discussion: Patient's possible manipulation of system. Could have queried appointment with practice before attending. Distress felt by doctors unable to help patients in pain because of long waiting lists and possible ways of having patients seen more quickly. For example, telephoning consultant direct and involvement of local Member of Parliament. Clarification of requested referral at consultation.

Decision: No decision as partner unable to attend meeting.

161. Wrong advice from hospital on baby's diet

Mother very depressed after each of three births. Baby ill and admitted with high temperature. Chest infection diagnosed and treated with antibiotics. Weighed in hospital and mother informed by nurses that baby was 2 kg overweight for age (2 months). Mother very upset and suffered relapse of depression. Put baby on diet. Partner informed her everything normal and weight right for height. Depression settled again in 2/3 weeks. Letter written to paediatric liaison health visitor expressing concern at anguish caused. No reply to date.

Discussion: Centile charts and parental trends of height and weight. Care in information given to parents.

Decision: To write again with copies to hospital consultant concerned and nursing manager requesting reply justifying information given.

162. Dopamine antagonists

Terminally ill patient presented with vomiting. Reason unknown. Given two dopamine antagonists, which caused patient to feel very ill.

Discussion: Leaflet given to all doctors on care of the dying. Photocopied list of different causes of vomiting handed out to doctors and appropriate drug treatments discussed.

Decision: No decision.

163. Prescribed amoxycillin: allergic

Presented with allergic rash. Mistake made nine days previously when patient presented with otitis media. Partner discovered allergy on notes and changed to another drug but not before computer passed amoxycillin through to dispensary.

Discussion: Prompting on computer screen.

Decision: To ask member of staff to raise issue with computer company on possibility of entry for drug allergy and prescribing.

164. Dermatomyositis

Included in list as a very rare diagnosis of interest. Female patient aged 40 presented with rash, very unwell, pain in wrists, puffy discoloured eyes and finger nails. Diagnosis missed at practice but referred to consultant immediately who then diagnosed.

Discussion: Diagnosis of this rare condition.

Decision: No decision.

165. Psoriasis

Female patient aged 72 with extremely bad psoriasis since childhood. Recent visit to homoeopath and given three tablets producing cure within one month.

Discussion: Significance with regard to conventional medicine. Nurses feel only relevant if patient is positive in belief. Other known homoeopathic doctors in area. Possibility of follow-up.

Decision: Partner to discuss matter with homoeopathic doctor involved and possibly invite to primary health care meeting.

166. Low haemoglobin: demented

Female patient aged 87 living in nursing home. Demented. Unable to recognize people but happy. Very pale and unsteady. Blood tests showed iron deficient but no other symptoms. Given iron and re-checked in one month. No better. Problem as to whether to undertake further investigations. Family declined on patient's behalf. Patient now has abdominal pain, is anorexic and fading. Colonic malignancy suspected but no diagnosis confirmed.

Discussion: Possibility of cause being curable if diagnosed but felt to be unlikely. Unlikelihood of patient having sufficient strength to withstand treatment if referred. Quality of life if prolonged. Wishes of relatives. Partner's unease at non-diagnosis. Necessity or otherwise for diagnosis to be confirmed in elderly patients.

Decision: It was agreed that partner concerned had acted correctly in abiding by wishes of relatives to do nothing further by way of investigations.

167. Low haemoglobin: 16+ check

History of heart problem. Follow-up at hospital. At 16+ check, tired, nails splitting and flaking. Haemoglobin checked 6.8 and no detectable ferritin. Mother has iron deficiency anaemia. Referred to haematologist for iron absorption tests. Considered to have no link with cardiac state.

Discussion: As above.

Decision: No decision.

168. Alcoholism

Male patient aged 48 drinking excessively and had disappeared. Wife asked practice for help. Partner telephoned police but patient returned voluntarily next day. Patient attended practice three weeks later shaking, sweating and feeling ill. Told he had 'alcohol withdrawal symptoms' and should be admitted for treatment. Considerable time taken in trying to find unit willing to accept patient, who then said he felt better and would handle at home. Partner felt opportunity lost.

Discussion: Difficulty in arranging admission to therapy unit. Friction in family and wife's refusal to accept therapy although felt she would derive support from relative support scheme. Role of community psychiatric nurse. General lack of psychiatric services in area. Family rather than patient seeking help. Daughter developing problems with anorexia and persistent urinary tract infections. Police involvement by partner.

Decision: The practice to offer assistance only when patient concerned actively seeks help and is prepared to confront problem. Not to breach confidentiality by involving police through information from third party.

169. Wound breakdown

Breast lump excised. Sutures removed after a week. Despite having been warned not to over-stretch, wound opened.

Discussion: Length of time for sutures depending on site.

Decision: To remind nurses to leave sutures for 10 days unless on face.

170. Dysuria: time lag in obtaining results

Female patient presented with cystitis for three days. Given sodium bicarbonate and a midstream urine specimen sent to laboratory. Patient returned three days later very uncomfortable. Very angry with lack of treatment. Given Monotrim and settled in 24 hours. Midstream urine result showed contaminants only.

Discussion: Management of dysuria. Practice protocol and difficulties involved as each case variable and needs treating accordingly. Merits of antibiotic therapy and dangers of prescribing antibiotics unnecessarily with possible medico-legal implications. Urine testing in practice and savings produced in time and money.

Decision: Practice manager to investigate midstream urine kits and costings. To have practice protocol for treating urine infections particularly in female patients but not to include overall antibiotic cover.

171. Deaf, dumb and blind patient: communication problem

Hospital telephoned practice to say patient admitted. Very ill. Suggested husband should attend. Husband also deaf and dumb—difficulty in communication. Nothing in notes regarding daughter's married name and address or any other relative or carer.

Discussion: Lack of relevant information in notes about relatives or carer and future procedure. Member of staff indicated wish to learn sign language. Possible teachers and courses available.

Decision: To record next of kin or carer at elderly health checks. To keep names, addresses and telephone numbers of relatives or carers updated on computer and notes. To investigate possibility of two members of staff learning sign language.

172. Collapse during minor surgery

Male patient aged 68 known epileptic. Minor surgery to right eye lid. Given local anaesthetic which caused bruising. Patient said felt faint and thought he was going to have fit. Eventually recovered.

Discussion: Advisory leaflet for patients before minor surgery regarding meals etc. Emergency equipment. Allowance time for recovery. Timing of minor surgery sessions and to allocate a specific period in week/month rather than fitting in to general surgery hours.

Decision: To look at more efficient use of time for minor surgery sessions.

173. Prescription for rabies vaccine: difficulty sorting out immunization schedule

Patient very angry at having to pay for malaria tablets after having been given rabies vaccine. Five-minute appointment took half an hour to sort out. Difficulty with injections. Had first. Did not want second.

Discussion: Practice policy for giving foreign travel vaccinations and payment. Referrals to British Airways for expensive exotic vaccinations which cannot be bought in single doses. Letter from Department of Health. Unclear advice. Single dose rabies vaccine and possibility of practice manager buying in. Protocols in each treatment room.

Decision: To review list of vaccinations and protocols on exotic vaccines.

174. Angina patient drowned

Postmortem revealed this 60-year-old patient had drowned at the swimming baths. He had a previous history of anginal type pains. He was seen by a consultant and treated with aspirin and beta blockers. Did not take medication on a regular basis. He denied he had an illness.

Discussion: Difficulties in dealing with such situations. It was thought to be possibly a communication problem. Presented with a cough, complained that his angina was worse and asked to be put back on medication. He was given a sick note and asked to come back in ten days. He did not return. This patient would not co-operate and denied his illness. It was acknowledged by all that some personalities just do not co-operate and there is little that can be done for them.

Decision: No decision.

175. Patient found to have angina: no previous cardiovascular screening

This 52-year-old patient had a previous history of hypertension which was well controlled on atenolol. She developed symptoms of tiredness and ankle swelling. Blood pressure was raised at this point but with treatment settled to 150/80. She also complained of chest pain and was sent for an exercise test after which she was diagnosed as having angina. She was a non-smoker, cholesterol 4, on hormone replacement therapy and had no family history of heart disease.

Discussion: On scanning notes for risk factors, it was found that this patient had not been invited for cardiovascular screening. Various reasons were offered as to why she had not been sent for, but it was acknowledged that it was important that screening must be targeted at risk groups. Meeting arranged to discuss banding for groups to be included and, also to see if the local FHSA's computer can be expanded to include those of the population at risk. Until that meeting there is little point in discussing how banding will affect which patients are called for cardiovascular screening.

Decision: None taken.

176. Patient admitted to hospital bleeding after minor operation: on anticoagulants

55-year-old patient with mitral valve replacement on anti-coagulants. Persuaded doctor to remove small lump below left eyebrow. Clotting time checked. Some concern about the risk of bacterial endocarditis. Persuaded against better judgement. Minor operation went well, but bleeding continued even after 45 minutes' pressure and ice. Patient admitted and treated. Good scar, pleased with the result.

Discussion: As above.

Decision: Not to allow patients to sway you against your own better judgement.

177. Mumps in a previously immunized child

Swelling in parotid area not vaccine associated. Child immunized five months previously.

Discussion: There was no way of preventing this happening. Lessons learned, vaccines are not 100% effective.

Decision: No decision.

APPENDIX 4

Administrative significant events discussed in audit meetings

1. Dissatisfied patient: referral

Male patient with history of dysuria and haematuria. Referred. Biopsy undertaken but no prostatic tissue taken. Further investigation refused. Patient complained of incompetence on part of hospital and practice for wrong referral. After consultation with Medical Defence Union, partner suggested change of doctor. No reply.

Discussion: As above and possible follow-up letter to patient.

Decision: To check with FHSA if patient has changed to another practice.

2. Further discussion, dissatisfied patient above

Following above complaint, partner said would re-refer should patient present with same symptoms. Hospital consultant supports registrar in handling of biopsy. Patient not taking matter further and has been seen at surgery on a regular basis.

Discussion: As above.

Decision: No further decision at present.

3. Patient complaint: nebulizer

Patient very angry about hospital nebulizer not working satisfactorily. Telephoned surgery and abusive to staff. Partner wrote to patient suggesting change of practice if not satisfied. Wife subsequently telephoned to apologise but no response from patient.

Discussion: As above.

Decision: No decision.

4. Patient complaint: test results

Aggressive businessman. Presented gastro-enteritis. Results showed salmonella. Partner on holiday. Patient not told result and annoyed. Department of Public Health informed, who visited house and did further tests. Adult son and daughter away and patient advised to bring them back. Patient still not informed of further test results and heard tests positive from friend at Department of Public Health (DPH).

Discussion: Grey area in system of telling patients of abnormal results which may be missed when patients expected to ring in. Doctor instigating tests should inform patient of result. Holiday cover and tightening up of procedures at surgery. Role of Department of Public Health in visiting homes without identification and their general policy in advising the public on hygiene.

Decision: To write to DPH for information on what advice is being given to patients and their protocol for dealing with salmonella infection. To tighten up areas for the giving of results and holiday cover.

5. Patient complaint: status asthmaticus

Visit requested. Doctor arrived 45 minutes later to find patient sweating, pulse high, using nebulizer. Wife had called 999 ambulance. Admitted. No sign of urgency in initial telephone call. Doctor had no injectable drug available but administered hydrocortisone. Visited on patient's return home. Complained about delay at first visit.

Discussion: Character of patient and wife. State of urgency. Why status developed. General discussion on steroid therapy.

Decision: Asthma calls to be visited immediately. Patients told to dial 999 *and* call surgery. More questions to be asked on the telephone to assess urgency. Steroid therapy should be 30 mg a day for 10 days. Patient should be seen a few days before end of course to assess and establish tailing off. Peak flow graph to be done by patient and brought with them to consultation.

6. Patient complaint: poor service

Difficult patient, not happy with diagnosis. Difficulty with insurance forms. Difficulty with repeat prescription. Patient telephoned practice manager very late at night at her home very angry.

Discussion: Dealing with insurance forms. Telephone calls to private homes. Relationship of reception staff with this particular family.

Decision: Insurance forms to be read more carefully. Patients to be made aware of regulations with regard to insurance forms, particularly if they wish to see them within the 21 days stipulated. No home phone numbers to be given out. Practice number to be used which will then be passed to duty doctor out of hours. A letter to be written to patient when there is a difficulty, rather than telephone call.

7. Patient complaint: reception

Patient felt reception staff could be more sympathetic.

Discussion: Patient's character. Felt to be a worrier. Reception staff telephone manners. Felt to be occasional sharpness.

Decision: Practice manager was aware and would look out for this, having a word if necessary.

8. Patient complaint: computer entry

Male patient attended for tetanus vaccination. Nurse checking computer record brought up 'alcohol problems'. Patient angry that everyone in practice had access and wanted it deleted as he said he had long since lost the problem.

Discussion: Need for pertinent information to be available and placed in records. Care to be taken always to switch off screen after each patient.

Decision: For entry to be moved over to 'Past Medical History' on computer.

9. Patient complaint: NHS

Female patient aged 79 full of grumbles and complaints over drug treatments and not being able to talk to partner on telephone. Asked for five-minute appointment before surgery began. Took half an hour to sort out causing late surgery. Seen in nurses' room. Very uncomfortable.

Discussion: Timing. Felt to be all right to see patient before surgery if quick. Improving facilities in nurses' room. System for dealing with complaints against practice. Problems for receptionist in ascertaining urgency and necessity for slipping patients in without appointments. Manipulative patients.

Decision: Receptionists to tell patients being seen before surgery that appointments begin at 9 a.m. and for doctor to endorse five-minute time limit on greeting patient. For appropriate furniture and equipment to be installed in nurses' room.

10. Patient complaint

Patient telephoned for prescription and, when told it would take 24 hours, he became abusive. The receptionist put the phone down on him. After the event a doctor wrote to the patient stating that there was no need to be abusive and if he was dissatisfied he could change practices. The patient replied stating his case. A letter of reply was sent by the practice manager explaining the situation and stating that the patient could stay with the practice if he wished.

Discussion: As above.

Decision: Staff told to pass over any problem they cannot handle diplomatically to another member of staff. This will help to diffuse a potentially tense situation and promote better staff-patient relations.

11. Patient complaint

Patient telephoned for a prescription late in the afternoon and told by one of the receptionists that he should have rung earlier. Patient then called the doctor out after abuse to the receptionist.

Discussion: Staff attitudes. It was concluded that staff should be more flexible in their attitude towards patients. At present their rigid attitude served only to antagonize patients.

Decision: Staff training through role play teaching how to handle tense situations more positively.

12. Demand to see notes

Very demanding couple who visit practice frequently with much minor illness. Patient very angry after gynaecological hospital visit. Read notes left in hospital waiting room and upset by referral letter written by partner to consultant mentioning overdose many years ago and personality disorder. Felt consultant's attitude affected by this and not relevant information. Patient saw different partner and demanded to see medical records and an explanation of style of letter writing. Patient asked to return when new Act had been checked and hospital telephoned for explanation. Copies of notes given to patient only from November last.

Discussion: The new Act and implications—a solicitor's letter and court order would be required for information before November. Referral letter writing styles and relevant content. Summary card content. Different consultants' attitudes and handling of patients. Behaviour of partners prior to referral—felt to have behaved impeccably in treatment offered. General rudeness of some patients and dealing with such.

Decision: Nothing further at present but to await outcome.

13. Request for medical records

Female patient aged 24 had pituitary tumour removed whilst registered with another practice. Emergency admission and patient considering legal action against previous general practitioner and requested records. Partner concerned out of practice and, despite being offered appointment on partner's return, patient refused and was very persistent. Reception staff agreed to copy notes but said doctor must be seen before released to patient. Notes released after changeover of staff.

Discussion: New Act which states patients have right to access to records from November 1991 with general practitioner's consent. Conveying urgency through staff changeovers. Patient advised by solicitor to obtain copies of notes—possible complaint to Law Society. Manipulation of staff by patient and alternative courses of action. Future action.

Decision: Patient must speak to doctor registered with or, if absent, a colleague to obtain permission to have copy of records. To see such patients at a private appointment after normal surgery hours and make a charge. No photocopying to be undertaken by secretaries unless authorized.

14. Patient complaint: drugs wrongly dispensed

Computer issued drugs not ordered—repeat prescription requested but not picked up some time ago. Patient received these as well as ones requested previous day. Very rude to practice manager.

Discussion: System for dealing with prescriptions not collected.

Decision: Check system. Check shelves every two months and put any left drugs back into stock. Contact patient to find out why not collected.

15. Registration of family from outside area

Family related to patients registered with practice. Dissatisfied with present practice and others in immediate area either full or not interested.

Discussion: Problems of this family and the possible reasons for them wishing to leave their present practice and being unable to find another willing to take them on to their list. Patients who move out of area but wish to remain on list. Patients who wish to be admitted to list but live outside area. Reception staff dealing with requests. Call-outs, particularly at night, when long distances are involved.

Decision: To tighten up boundaries and make policy decision at next practice meeting. To be more strict where town visiting may be necessary. For patients to be advised to remain with present practice until a decision has been made at practice meeting as to whether they will be accepted or not depending on location and any other special circumstances. To see as temporary patient if recently moved and no general practitioner but out of practice area, and to try to persuade patient to seek a closer practice.

16. Change of practice request

Aggressive and difficult patient asked by another practice in area to find new practice. Practice not informed of likelihood of patient registering.

Discussion: Protection of staff from abuse by patients. Removal from list if necessary.

Decision: No decision at present time.

17. Change of practice request

Female patient aged 40 expressed dissatisfaction with another practice in area. Requested transfer because not happy with treatment. Not much past medical history apparent when questioned other than a little arthritis. On arrival, medical records showed psychiatric problems + + with many referrals and treatments.

Discussion: Difficulties sometimes experienced by doctor in assessing patients who request transfer and have unrealistic expectations. Ways of limiting input and time spent in consultation after constant failure. Partners sometimes in favour of having fresh start between partners within practice.

Decision: To try to persuade patients not being realistic about their problems to remain with present practice and to point out possible delays involved with starting treatment again. To have right of refusal if dissatisfied with reasons for wanting change.

18. Stealing

Girl aged 12 from family of 4 children. Mother blind, father congenital palsy. Would not talk in front of parents and partner suggested patient should return on own. Did not happen and parents have not sought further advice.

Discussion: Responsibility of practice in preventing possible chronic problem. Use of health visitor and other possible approaches to family.

Decision: Partner to talk to health visitor and possibly telephone family to offer help. To have immediate follow-up with any further problem.

19. Abuse to district nurse

Female patient with ongoing leg ulcers and maggots. Very abusive and aggressive over a long period. Partner informed patient that if she continued she must find another practice. Patient apologized and manner improved.

Discussion: Accepting difficult patients from other practices and FHSA rules of allocation as last resort. Courtesy telephone call to other practice likely to take patient.

Decision: No decision.

20. Request for oral contraception during son's appointment

Mother told at reception to ask for repeat prescription during son's consultation.

Discussion: Necessity of following contraception protocol and regular checks required. Manipulation of receptionists and abuse of appointment system.

Decision: To educate patients about practice rules concerning appointments and to ask them to comply in future. For reception staff to ask doctor first if they will see patient and send up notes. Article to be put in Patients Participation Group magazine.

21. Anger about wife changing daughter's name

Divorced parents. Mother changed back to maiden name and wanted daughter's name changed on medical records. Father found out at school and very upset.

Discussion: Legal position. At present, parent with care and control has right to access to confidential information. Other parent must apply to court. Medical records not a legal document and patient can change name on these. Role of reception. Other similar cases involving name changes and difficulties involved.

Decision: Receptionists not to be involved in such cases but to refer directly to a doctor. No confidential information to be given out in reception. To clarify legal situation with regard to new Act.

22. Insulin dispensing error

Patient worried about insulin received and telephoned early morning to ask advice. Advised to take same dose as usual before going to work and bring drugs to surgery for checking. Patient rang again after injecting drug. Completely wrong combination given resulting in 6 × normal dose. Advised to

go immediately to casualty before becoming hypoglycaemic. Admitted and stabilized.

Discussion: Differences in types of insulin and necessary dosage changes. Error checked back. Order correct. Distributed wrongly although invoiced correctly by supplier. Not double checked by dispenser. Supplier unable to send correct drug for two days.

Decision: To remove drug from bag and show to patient for confirmation before handing over. If collected by another person, to ask for drug to be checked before use. To be put on agenda for next staff meeting.

23. Wrong drug dispensed

Discussion: Discussed at time of incident.

Decision: No further decision.

24. Dispensing errors

Drugs wrongly dispensed owing to 'pressure of work'. Incidence book set up. Random mistakes from different staff.

Discussion: Dispensing methods and safety techniques, particularly checking. Staff in dispensary: 1 at hatch; 1 on phone; 1 dispensing. Telephone to be transferred to practice manager when single member of staff in dispensary.

Decision: Practice manager to report back to staff saying doctors very upset. Safety measures not adhered to and general procedure to be tightened up, particularly checking system. Double checking will be introduced if mistakes continue to be made over next three months. Half used packets of drugs must be left in box and marked. Prescriptions to stay in bag with script until handed over to patient.

25. Dispensing error by receptionist

Drug checked by two receptionists.

Discussion: Dispensing. Not felt to be sensible to be using receptionists together when training dispensers.

Decision: Only time receptionists will dispense is after 7 p.m. or Saturday morning when doctor/nurse will check. Patients to be asked to wait when dispensers having coffee breaks, etc.

26. Falsification of prescription by patient

Twenty-year old patient with a history of bulimia, alcohol and drug abuse for which she was being treated by a psychiatrist. Complained of not sleeping, given advice on relaxation but said this did not work. Came to see general practitioner saying psychiatrist had told her to come to see him for a prescription for sleeping tablets. There was no accompanying letter. General practitioner very dubious about prescribing but allowed her 10 Welldorm tablets on prescription in both words and number. Twenty minutes later, chemist phoned to say the prescription had been altered to 30 capsules and asked for clarification. It was decided not to inform the police. Another appointment was made for the patient but not kept.

Discussion: The point was raised with reference to other forms that are forged, for example FW8 used to gain housing points.

Decision: All forms to be written in words and number. Any alterations to be signed.

27. Prescription request by telephone: no record

Patient visited with allergic reaction to something requested for cough over telephone and not written in notes. Partner did not know what had been prescribed.

Discussion: As above.

Decision: To pull notes after telephone calls and record details.

28. Hib given instead of flu vaccination

Partner in hurry took wrong box from refrigerator and administered wrong vaccine.

Discussion: Checking system as in hospitals. Clearer packaging and possible approach to manufacturers. Recording on computer before giving as extra check. Temperature of vaccines.

Decision: To have discussion with nurses on avoidance of mistakes by double-checking and clearer labelling in refrigerator.

29. Flu vaccine given instead of tetanus

Patient given appointment in middle of flu vaccine clinic for booster tetanus injection. Mistake made and came to light following week when patient saw partner with cut finger.

Discussion: High proportion of nurses' time doing clerical work. Realistic procedure time allocation. Need to employ another nurse, adequate profile of person to be employed and training of such person. Audit of nurse time before employing new nurse.

Decision: Nursing time audit to be done and, in particular, how many patients referred without appointment to nurses during surgery hours. To ask patients to make future appointment to see nurses rather than be seen immediately. Meeting set up to discuss ideas with nurses. Aims and criteria list to be produced.

30. Meningitis vaccine

Nurses voiced concern over future payments for this vaccine.

Discussion: Partial reimbursement. Vaccination of under 4s and future targets. Injection cards. Holiday vaccinations and payments. Hepatitis B vaccinations and unsuccessful groups of patients.

Decision: Stated partner to draw up protocol for travel vaccinations generally.

31. Efcortelan in nurses' room out of date

Patient with anaphylactic reaction. Doctor found drug two months out of date. Nurses reported that situation rectified immediately.

Discussion: Disposal of dangerous drugs. Responsibility of partners for disposal of unused drugs. Tightening up of procedures for checking expiry dates of drugs.

Decision: To check expiry date of drugs on delivery. To check drugs kept on premises once a month. To tighten up procedure for disposal of discarded drugs and in particular dangerous drugs such as MST.

32. Resistance to erythromycin

Telephoned by bacteriologist concerning evidence of resistance to erythromycin and advised to use penicillin where necessary.

Discussion: Excellent liaison with Bacteriology Department which keeps practice well informed. Patient with salmonella at local nursing home.

Decision: As advised, to use penicillin where appropriate.

33. Fisherman collapsed: heart attack protocol

Event already discussed at a previous meeting but anxiety expressed by partners on new protocol relating to receptionists advising patients over the telephone to take aspirin in suspected cases of heart attack while waiting for doctor and ambulance to arrive.

Discussion: Contra-indications for taking of aspirin, for example ulcers. Advice to be given by receptionist staff and calling ambulance for patient as a kindness to relatives.

Decision: To discuss matter further with regional medical adviser. Reception to ask if ambulance been called and, if not, to do so. To tell patient doctor will be contacted if not in building and will attend as quickly as possible. For reception staff not to advise patient to take aspirin but to wait and be given by doctor. To be discussed at next staff meeting.

34. Practice policy on appointment system

Difficulty in fitting in 'same day' appointments. Partners have different preferences as to seeing extras.

Discussion: Practice policy for the future. Falling numbers and existing competitive situation.

Decision: Protocols decided upon to meet each individual doctor's preference about seeing extra patients when appointment lists are full. Clause to be inserted in all contracts outlining policy on urgent appointments. Surgery hours to be extended if the need is there.

35. Digoxin audit

VTS mini audit. Trainee reported little recording of pulse readings at practice. Recording criteria arrived at by other trainees not particularly agreed with by partners.

Discussion: As above.

Decision: Better recording of pulse rate. To discuss at clinical meeting.

36. At risk groups: protocol

Two homosexual patients seen by nurses. No notes available or information on computer regarding possible positive HIV. Nurses worried by absence of information and felt protocol needed for treatment room as they may be compromising care of other patients. Asked for 'right to know' if doctors aware.

Discussion: Confidentiality aspect of unproven suspicions in notes and computer. Flagging system. Treatment room procedure and wearing of gloves. Staff precautions.

Decision: A positive HIV result is a clinical event and will be recorded as such in notes and on computer. Patients in the 'at risk' group will not necessarily have details recorded to limit any unnecessary slur. For staff to be alert and cautious when treating patients but to treat everyone in same way with maximum care against infection.

37. and 38. Two separate cases of elderly patients at risk: discussed under one heading

First patient an elderly gentleman living on his own, frail and in poor housing. Has been visited regularly over three years but refuses entry into house. Neighbours concerned about him falling over and persuaded eventually to go to casualty for treatment. Still declining offers of help.

The second patient has paranoiac psychosis but despite this manages to look after herself and keep herself clean. Not ill enough to section despite pressure from family to do so. It was considered best to leave her while she is coping.

Discussion: As above.

Decision: An 'at risk' register to be drawn up to include patients who are seriously at risk. More discussion on which risk categories to include. Guidelines on type of help to be given to these patients.

39. Visit request not done

Request telephoned in but not put in book. Doctor forgot during surgery until patient phoned again and doctor was able to visit in evening. Excessive and continuous pain. Difficulty in diagnosis.

Discussion: Patient complaints generally. This particular patient's late referral and diagnosis. Patient's personality in view of persistent complaints. Test results not always being available in notes.

Decision: Doctor involved should make visit soon after complaint to deflate situation by discussion with patient. Test results should be known to all doctors when care shared.

40. Accident call-out: severe disruption to surgery

Patient dived into swimming-pool and fractured spine. Partner called by ambulance service. Flying squad took one and a half hours to come. No other partner to take evening surgery. Patients notified and offered other appointments.

Discussion: Problems of small practice when partner called out and no other partners to cover.

Decision: No decision.

41. Telephone not properly transferred

Wrong tape inserted into machine when surgery closed. Unlikely to recur.

Discussion: As above.

Decision: No decision.

42. Branch surgery improvements

Improvement grant requested for surgery in developing rural village with little public transport and growing population of elderly and young families. The need to keep open was questioned in reply and that costs would not make this a feasible proposition.

Discussion: Number of patients using service who are unable to attend main practice and call-outs involved. Distribution of medicines by local post office. Patient questionnaire to assess needs. Possible loss of patients to other practices in area should surgery close. Parish Council letter supporting proposals.

Decision: To pass on positive results of survey together with letter from Parish Council for further consideration.

43. Surgery building

Attempted break-in. Trouble with drains.

Discussion: System for dealing with problems. Workmen who would be prepared to give immediate attention and to work out of hours if necessary. Security and further protection of building.

Decision: To compile a comprehensive list of local workmen who could deal with matters such as burglar alarm, plumbing, replacing windows.

44. Blanket burn from lamp

Nurse found examination lamp left on and touching blanket causing scorch mark.

Discussion: As above and possibility of fire.

Decision: All lamps to be unplugged at night.

45. Trainee on duty alone

Discussion: As above.

Decision: Always accompany trainee for first three months.

46. Only two doctors working: one called out

Appointment system looked at. Minimum of 50 appointment slots per day needed plus open access. Working well for a month but cannot legislate for the unusual. Above situation will be eradicated using locums where necessary.

Discussion: As above.

Decision: No further decision.

47. Two rota changes leaving only one doctor on open access morning surgery

One doctor available who saw 31 patients in open surgery session.

Discussion: Workable rotas and need for more than one doctor to be available in case of call-out. Receptionist to monitor appointment book and check changes to rotas, etc.

Decision: Matter to be discussed at later date.

48. Rota changes

Discussion: Handover policy when going off duty.

Decision: A positive handover with doctor going off duty ringing through personally to hand over.

49. Case conference

Girl aged 13—? sexually abused by 17-year-old. Mother worried about antisocial behaviour, for example stealing. Father RAF and worried about career if social services brought in. Child had been on 'at risk' register aged 3—mother worried about violent feelings towards daughter.

Discussion: Family therapy/child guidance. Mother seen but father refused to take part. Nothing done. Family relationships discussed. Use of health visitor. Confidentiality aspect and legal requirements. Team approach within health centre. Primary health care meeting as forum for discussion. Other agencies which may be of help.

Decision: Confidentiality aspect to be discussed at next practice primary health care meeting. Social worker to go back to family and try to persuade them gently towards therapy.

50. Talk on hormone replacement therapy: no nurse present

Nurses concerned that a nurse should be present for further questions and debriefing after talk. Considered to be a good time for health education.

Discussion: Further talks with nurses to work out appropriate format. Success of hormone replacement therapy clinic. Possibility of other partners being trained.

Decision: Subgroup to discuss further number and timing of hormone replacement therapy clinics.

51. Lack of liaison between health care professionals

Patient with terminal carcinoma lung sent home by hospital. Required general nursing and support from district nurses, who were not told Macmillan nurse also visiting. Confusion for patient's wife over care instructions.

Discussion: General liaison with outside health care professionals.

Decision: To invite Macmillan nurse to specific case meetings in future to avoid difficulties and unpleasantness.

52. Failure of communication: nurses

Patients changing doctor after change of partnership were required to attend for checks. Letters sent without knowledge of nurses.

Discussion: As above.

Decision: Copy of all letters calling patients in for checks to be given to doctors and nurses. Primary health care meetings to start shortly with nurses and health visitors present.

53. Leak of confidential information

Woman patient in her mid-30s wished to discuss contraception and the use of coil. Had only discussed with partner. Friend subsequently mentioned it to patient. Appointment made verbally over the telephone. Not known how leak occurred but it has to be assumed that the book was seen.

Discussion: Possible areas where such a leak could happen. Tightening up of system for the future.

Decision: No names to be said out loud when making telephone appointments for confidential matters. To use codes in the appointment book for such matters, as initials such as IUCD are often understood by patients. The appointment book and lists in nurses' room not to be too visible. Private hatch to be used if confidential matter to be discussed when making appointment.

54. Information given over the telephone

Information given to somebody posing as a patient when in fact she was an impostor. Phone call received asking for results of investigations. Ten minutes later, person rang anonymously to say that the first caller was an impostor.

Discussion: As above.

Decision: Potentially damaging information to be given in person and not over telephone.

55. Confidentiality

Nursing officer phoned to enquire about one of her nursing staff who was a patient at the practice. On the first occasion, she telephoned to ask if the patient had an appointment the next day and had been issued with a sick note. The receptionist was not intimidated by her abrasive manner and reported the incident to a partner, who dealt with the matter and received an apology for the incident.

Discussion: Staff to be spoken to regarding confidentiality and be told that under no circumstances is information to be given out over the telephone.

Decision: As above.

56. Collapse: 999 call: no ambulance available

Partner called during surgery hours. Off-duty ambulance crew arrived 20 minutes later. Partner and staff responded correctly to call. Patient suffered cardiac arrest in presence of partner.

Discussion: Necessity of back-up ambulance crew to be available. Need for official complaint.

Decision: Short letter to health authority to mark situation.

57. Hospital discharge without instructions

Patient admitted for anal skin tag tidy up. Discharged with pack *in situ*. Patient had no instructions. District nurse rang ward to be told pack should have been removed previous day. Patient in great pain and doctor unable to examine properly. Felt to be very unsatisfactory.

Discussion: Hospital discharges and need for better instructions. Dissatisfaction with this particular surgical procedure.

Decision: Partner to write to hospital to voice complaint.

58. Hospital admission slip lost

Relative requested slip Saturday morning. Receptionist on own and had to leave reception to search but unable to find. Partner able to retrieve situation.

Discussion: Importance patients attach to having slip when being admitted, although rarely used. System for dealing with slips in practice and delays involved whilst in trays waiting for signature.

Decision: Nothing to be done except to warn patients that a delay is likely at weekends and, if necessary, to tell hospital that they have been unable to get a signature.

59. Letter sent: appointment not received

Patient complained that she had not received an appointment which should have been dealt with three months previously. There have been problems with this particular consultant's clinic in the past. After a letter was sent by the practice, the situation was rectified.

Discussion: As above.

Decision: Nothing to be done, but be aware of the situation with this particular consultant's appointment system.

60. Supply of tablets kept by hospital on discharge

Patient admitted for constipation and in hospital for two hours. Own tablets taken away and discharged with six-day supply only, despite repeat prescription from surgery on day of admission. Patient has difficulty in getting to surgery to collect drugs and likes to keep ample supply.

Discussion: Comparative systems at two hospitals with regard to patients' own drugs.

Decision: To write to therapeutics committee at hospital involved with regard to patients' own drugs. To ask for situation to be reviewed and a policy statement for patients to be returned drugs they came in with.

61. Late arrival of ambulance to emergency call

Doctor made a 999 call for patient *in extremis*. Second call received to attend patient with asthma attack. Unable to leave first patient until ambulance arrived. Ambulance delayed by three quarters of an hour, the call having been accepted and transferred to another ambulance service but giving the wrong address.

Discussion: Potential serious situation arising and dilemma of divided responsibility for the doctor involved.

Decision: Letter to be sent to ambulance service to clarify which area is covered by them.

62. Pathology specimens not delivered to hospital

Partners felt this to be very serious misdemeanour needing to be dealt with at the time. Very off-hand member of staff. Blamed lapse on premenstrual tension. Partners unhappy at events as it affected doctors, staff and patients. Given first verbal warning as it showed complete lack of responsibility. Staff unhappy and question present arrangement for delivery of specimens.

Discussion: As above.

Decision: To continue with present arrangement for delivery of specimens. To give second warning if matters do not improve. Attend to premenstrual tension problem.

63. Patient not informed of hospital's request for change of medication

Discussion: Information to patient of change before pre-scription dispensed. Reception communication and handover period when important items outstanding.

Decision: To discuss communication problems at next primary health care meeting.

64. Missed referral

Patient 15 weeks pregnant. Missed writing referral letter.

Discussion: Writing referral letters during consultation.

Decision: For patients to be told to enquire if appointment not received from hospital within two weeks of consultation.

65. Missed referral

Discussion: Difficulty in remembering to refer after further discussion on other aspects during consultation.

Decision: To tell patients to return if they have not heard from the hospital within two/three weeks.

66. Missed referral

Discussion: To look in more detail at a method of seeing that referrals are not missed. The system relies mainly upon doctors putting notes onto correct piles in order that notes are not filed away. One suggestion was to check each set of notes at the end of each surgery.

Decision: More discussion needed, no decision.

67. Patient request for sight of report before posting: system failed

Patient very upset when found report to employers already posted after requesting sight thereof. Read copy and was satisfied.

Discussion: System failure between secretaries. Protocols in general.

Decision: Note sticking system worked out to prevent re-occurrence. Protocols started for all procedures. File in reception for gathering in administrative protocols.

68. Letter to reduce medication not acted upon

Consultant's letter advising reduction in medication was not acted upon.

Discussion: Reading letters more carefully. Marking 'action'. Draw notes and put in trays. Reception to re-direct if letter marked 'action' in filing. Clearer hospital letters. Patients being told of changes to treatments.

Decision: Practice manager to bring up subject of a clear 'action line' in hospital letters reporting on patients at next outpatient quality meeting and the need for patients to be told of any change to their treatment.

69. No letter after smear test

Result back negative. No letter sent to patient.

Discussion: Recall system on computer and letters sent out. System for positive results.

Decision: To talk to computer operator, who handles recall letters, at appropriate time. Stamped addressed envelopes for results to be added to invitation letter. Patients to be told to contact practice if not heard result within six weeks—to be inserted in invitation letter.

70. No death certificate available

Partner not available when relatives arrived from distance. Death occurred at night and arrangements transacted through social services control centre. Relatives already left home when doctor rang to say appointment made not convenient.

Discussion: Difficulty of arrangements transacted through third party. Visiting relatives at home to deliver death certificate. Discussed previously and new protocol working well except when third party involved. Direct access by telephone to mobile warden when necessary to obtain further information before a visit at night that has been requested by control room.

Decision: To leave all messages concerning death certificates at reception. To note direct access to mobile warden possible by telephone at night for further information, if necessary, before visit requested by control room.

71. Private certificates

Patient requiring second certificate for work purposes. Patient queried charge after not being charged on first occasion. Embarrassing situation. Partner felt practice inconsistent in management of fees and behaving irrationally.

Discussion: Practice policy with regard to charges for private treatment. Role of office and reception in handling requests and charges to take onus from doctors to make instant decisions during surgery hours. Education of patients with regard to charges and presenting and collecting forms.

Decision: To minimize form filling, if presented during consultations, by requesting form to be left for completion later. To educate patients to leave forms at reception for payment and completion. For reception to be explicit concerning collection at least 48 hours later. Practice consistency. List of charges to be circulated to all doctors and nurses. Details to be inserted in newsletter, new patient pack and posters in all waiting areas. Charges for yellow fever vaccinations to revert to being handled by reception.

72. Letter not written for urgent appointment

Letter was thought to have been written. All failsafe mechanisms failed.

Discussion: Still do not know how this happened. May have occurred before 'for action' stickers were in use. Need to review if situation recurs.

Decision: Monitor the situation but continue with present system until situation clarified.

73. Report received and not acted upon: urinary tract infection in a diabetic

A positive urine culture result on a diabetic patient was received but not acted upon. The patient had not been informed despite having telephoned to ask for a result.

Discussion: It was agreed by all partners that it was the responsibility of the person requesting the test to take action upon it. However, it was noted that this system could fall down on three counts, namely: if a locum requests a test, if a doctor goes away, or if a doctor is not in.

Decision: The doctor responsible for prescribing treatment is responsible for seeing that action is taken to ensure test results are acted upon and the patient is informed. "To start or going on" to be written in appropriate box on pathology forms so that laboratory know what antibiotics are being given.

74. Midstream urine sample report: needed treatment: signed by two doctors but not done

Two reports received. The first stating no significant growth and the second stating that a significant growth of haemolytic streptococcus had been identified. The second report was not seen until after the patient came in to pick up a prescription.

Discussion: As above.

Decision: Keep things as they are.

75. Note attached to patient's notes: health check not done

Patient rude, abusive and alcoholic.

Discussion: Difficult patients. If a health check is due, is offered by the doctors, then refused, there is nothing to be done.

Decision: System satisfactory. Patient awkward.

76. Two incidences of name changed on computer but not on records

Events occurred before protocol for this procedure put into use.

Discussion: As above.

Decision: Continue with protocol set.

77. Discharge not on computer

Patient discharged from hospital. Discharge summary not stamped.

Discussion: All laboratory reports come into surgery at lunch time, so all post is not seen or highlighted on the same day. Problems also arise when patients hand in letters personally.

Decision: Remind all staff that post needs to be stamped with date of receiving. A 'v' to be marked in letters if they are on computer. If letters are given into the surgery they must be initialled and put into the system.

78. Issued with nebulizer without patient being seen

Parents contacted practice and nebulizer issued. Familiar with usage.

Discussion: Seeing patients before issue. Steroid therapy for patients who require nebulizer. Advice sheet for handing out. Peak flow chart to be read over phone when requesting nebulizer. Cleaning and testing of nebulizers. Protocol for use and issue of nebulizers.

Decision: Protocol will be written by partner and trainee. When nebulizer booked out, number of machine to be noted for tracing. If out for more than two weeks, practice nurse to trace and call in for checking electrically and cleaning. Advice sheets to be obtained from Asthma Society.

79. Poor patient/doctor communication about blood tests

Patient given an appointment for fasting blood tests at evening surgery.

Discussion: Advice note for patients to make morning appointments if fasting required. General communication between doctor and patient.

Decision: No more written instructions to be issued but staff to be asked to remember to advise patients about fasting and time of appointments.

80. Wrong information given over the telephone about results

Female patient told lipids raised after initial test and would need repeat in a month. Now told original test well within target range.

Discussion: Interpretation of results.

Decision: To consider re-designing stamp for clearer help to non-medical staff. For doctors always to tick appropriate box as to whether normal or not. To exercise care with interpreting results as target ranges can be confusing.

81. New patient allocated to wrong doctor

Patient angry with treatment received from previous practice. Put on list of wrong partner for patient's area. Partner felt it to be important to make good contact at first consultation.

Discussion: Areas and patients allocated to individual partners. Four counties involved. Role of reception.

Decision: To re-define and tighten up allocation lists. To discuss further on appointment of new partner.

82. Positive smear result given to patient as negative

Patient telephoned for result four weeks after having smear test. Told smear result not back. Ten days later, patient contacted the surgery again and was told result negative. Shortly afterwards she was contacted by the FHSA. She telephoned the surgery and was informed that she had pre-cancerous cells. Result was followed up with a letter. The patient telephoned again and was given advice. She was also told to come in to see her doctor. Ten days after this conversation, the patient's mother rang to say that she was seeking advice from a solicitor about the treatment her daughter had received.

Discussion: As above.

Decision: Record on continuation sheet all advice given to patients awaiting results. Patients to be told if smear is not normal. Dates to be checked on smear results before giving out information. A letter to be sent to the patient detailing events and to be marked 'without prejudice'.

83. Patient in waiting room two hours

Discussion: Staff training time. Waiting room awareness. Monitoring flow of surgeries. Checking surgery boxes prior to surgery. Doctors' lists kept up to date by receptionists. Notice in waiting room telling patients to make themselves known if waiting for any length of time.

Decision: To sharpen up procedure at front desk. Receptionists to tell patients reason for delay and approximate length of waiting time.

84. Failure to attend clinic

Two patients booked into cryo-therapy clinic for minor surgery failed to attend depriving others on waiting list.

Discussion: Reminder letters. Charging fee and possibly not re-booking unless very good reason for absence. Information regarding procedure at clinic.

Decision: Leaflet to be given to patient when appointment made explaining procedure. Existing leaflet to be altered to advise patients, if necessary, to cancel well in advance.

85. Appointment availability

This is a recurring problem which gets worse if a doctor is away. Adjustments have been made to ameliorate the situation by switching from open to more booked surgeries. In the past there were three open to one booked surgery. At present there are two open to two booked surgeries. In future there will be one open to three booked surgeries.

Discussion: As above. It is hoped that this will help to sort out the problem of patients having to wait up to five days for an appointment with a particular doctor. Open surgeries are to be for emergencies only, reducing patients to a handful rather than the large numbers (up to seventy) that are seen at present.

Decision: Move from open to booked surgeries. Advise patients on changes.

86. Lack of appointment space

Female partner has different types of surgeries from other doctors in the practice: they tend to be for emotional, gynae-cological and children's problems; 90%–95% of her patients are female.

Discussion: The appointment system and workload in general. Ideas concerning longer surgery times and computerizing the appointments system were discussed as was altering the hor-mone replacement therapy clinic.

Decision: Audit repeat appointments. Set a time for booking surgeries in advance. Alter appointments for male doctors as well, so that their workload is spread more evenly through the week.

87. Emergency treatment: nursing appointments full

Female patient presented at desk with cut hand. Local chemist advised stitching. Both nurses fully booked. Patient sent to casualty. Practice manager in reception at time and not happy with situation.

Discussion: Advice felt to be not good enough and minimum treatment considered to be appropriate in such cases. Merits of individual cases and necessity to respond.

Decision: For nurse to reassure patient by seeing quickly even if busy with others. If nursing time full, patient to be seen by doctor if one on premises. Patient to be told doctor can accommodate and to wait quietly and patiently.

88. Failure to meet immunization target

Percentages worked out incorrectly. Correction completed.

Discussion: As above.

Decision: No decision.

89. Failure to meet immunization target

Difference in FHSA-assessed figures for preschool vaccinations and practice assessment.

Discussion: Computer entries incorrectly inserted giving false data.

Decision: Meeting to discuss computerization and the need for another terminal.

90. Non-identification of patient

Visit request by note left at branch surgery stating Christian name only. Practice unable to identify until hospital rang next day having admitted patient with fractured leg.

Discussion: Damage prevention to practice.

Decision: Hospital telephoned and asked to notify partner when patient discharged for an explanation visit.

91. Installation of 486 (computer)

Computer off air for seven working days. No contingency plans worked out beforehand as time factor not known. Staff upset.

Discussion: Contingency plans for future. Dealing with backlog and at what stage to begin handwriting prescriptions. Notes inadequate without computer, keeping up-to-date front sheet on notes and writing in present medications at consultations. Counterfoils put in notes. Access to records in event of break-down.

Decision: Practice manager to consider problem and produce guidelines for an alternative route to be implemented im-mediately on breakdown.

92. Financial problem

Partnership change and lack of liaison between solicitors and accountants.

Discussion: As above.

Decision: Future forward planning. Several solicitors and ac-countants to be approached on charges for future legal work.

93. Practice progress

Discussion: Course costings. Courses available for different staff members and possible FHSA re-imbursement if approved. Need to update regularly.

Decision: Practice will fund courses where considered necessary and partners felt courses on money management/computers often gave the practice considerable savings.

94. Patient had three inappropriate letters

Male patient attended diabetic clinic and received three letters following day requesting he attend for 'over 75' check, flu vaccine and blood tests. Very angry

Discussion: Letters going out and irritation caused if patient already had procedure offered. Information to patients about procedures received. Updating of computer with summaries.

Numbers of patients responding to letters and percentages of patients waiting to be called for certain procedures.

Decision: Priority to get all summaries on to the computer as soon as possible. Devise protocol for follow on. Clinical meeting and discussion with member of staff who will be responsible for system.

95. Not 'our' patient

Patient given number on arrival at reception for surgery and jumped queue to see doctor. Wrong notes found (same name). Patient no longer registered with practice but seen 2 days previously when same thing happened. Took three quarters of an hour to sort out. Urgent call-out straight after caused chaos.

Discussion: Mechanism for seeing each other's patients if necessary. Difficulties in reception over transferring patients to other partners if do not know what is happening. Communication between partners and reception. Emergency doctor primarily responsible for overflow, late visits and urgent call-outs.

Decision: Receptionists to ring through to doctor for information if aware that surgery is getting behind. Partners to ask for help from others if in difficulties with surgery.

96. Three incidences of standing room only in the waiting room

Discussion: Busy Monday evenings at 6 p.m. in particular and peak time overcrowding generally. It was suggested that receptionists need to note who is running behind and the time the last patient booked. A clearer picture would then arise as to which doctor is running behind and why.

Decision: Receptionist to log who is running behind time. Once this is established action can be taken.

97. Two incidences of standing room only in the waiting room

Still trying to find out why the first incident happened. The second was a result of two doctors being called out on emergency visits.

Discussion: There is nothing to be done about the waiting room being crowded if duty doctors are called out. It was noted that appointments are well spaced with patients rarely having to wait more than twenty minutes.

Decision: Nothing to be done if duty doctors are called out.

98. Four incidences of patients standing in waiting room

This has been discussed previously and a solution suggested, which unfortunately has not yet been implemented.

Discussion: Monday changes to system. It was thought that Wednesday appointments are usually satisfactory and no changes were necessary.

Decision: Two extra appointments are to be blocked on Mondays when surgery is most busy.

99. No seats available downstairs waiting room

Discussion: Patients can go upstairs but feel isolated. A call board was suggested but this was rejected. It was pointed out that it had been used before to little avail. The call system works reasonably well, and the situation will be better with more booked surgeries.

Decision: To leave system alone. No decision.

100. Notes misfiled

Rheumatology test results entered on son's notes by mistake.

Discussion: As above.

Decision: No decision.

101. Notes misfiled

Letter in wrong notes. Check revealed no similarities or co-incidences between notes.

Discussion: Possible confusion due to one patient being temporary resident. Methods of filing and clipping letters together.

Decision: To file temporary resident notes separately in envelopes clearly marked T/R.

102. Notes misfiled

Notes put in wrong envelope by doctor. Some missing.

Discussion: As above.

Decision: To alert all members of staff.

103. Notes misfiled

Notes in wrong envelope. Two patients seen by two different doctors on different dates.

Discussion: Teaching sessions with trainee. Referrals. Any similarities.

Decision: No decision—a mistake.

104. TSH/T4 result not on computer

Retired general practitioner aged 65. Diagnosed myxoedema. Very insistent on regular blood tests to include thyroid stimulating hormone (TSH) every time as well as thyroxine estimation (T4). On two occasions partner unable to locate TSH results. Wrongly told patient result satisfactory.

Discussion: Necessity to rationalize processing of results from path. lab. and need to improve turnover with regard to computer and receptionists as embarrassment caused when patient arrives and no results available.

Decision: Working party to hold meeting to discuss system requirements for processing of results with view to functioning more efficiently. To advise necessary modifications to present complicated system and assess priorities. Suggestions in writing in 1 month from each branch of staff.

105. Wrong address on records

Patient in a nursing home now. Change not put on to records. Doctor wasted 20 minutes trying to find out where this patient was.

Discussion: As above.

Decision: To reinforce the message that changes of address are noted and recorded.

106. Information requested on AIDS

Information requested in reception. Duty receptionist shouted request across reception. Patient apparently unaware.

Discussion: Confidentiality. Staff procedure. Queue at windows, particularly bringing and collecting of prescriptions.

Decision: Nothing further on confidentiality aspect. Practice manager spoken to staff. To have further discussion on prescription handling and need for separate queues. Possibly to extend space for this purpose.

107. Surfeit of training

Felt to be too much in short space of time and surgeries left short because people training. Not felt to have been planned efficiently. Some courses felt to be inappropriate by doctors.

Discussion: Courses available to fulfil FHSA requirements. Needs of individual staff and thinking ahead for coming year. Even spread of postgraduate courses throughout five-year period.

Decision: Stated partner to work out structure for postgraduate courses over five-year period and to discuss plans periodically.

108. Police return stolen sick note pad

Found on housing estate. Did not know missing. General lapse in habit of locking pads up. Could have been used for defrauding social security.

Discussion: As above.

Decision: To be more vigilant, tighten up security and lock pads away at end of day.

109. Police call

Call to certify death during busy Saturday morning surgery. Partner away from surgery for 30 minutes leaving one receptionist only in very vulnerable position.

Discussion: Large Saturday morning surgeries, control of numbers attending and need for further receptionist. Worry concerning longer call-outs, being police surgeons, and need for extra medical back-up.

Decision: Another doctor to be on call and available if necessary. To consider budget aspects of a second receptionist/ practice nurse for Saturday morning surgery.

APPENDIX 5

The conventional audits

The audits undertaken by the 10 practices in the conventional audit arm of the study are listed below. (Each undertook six audits over a year, of which the first two were to concern diabetes mellitus and the appointments system; the other four were discretionary.)

1. Clinical

1–10	Diabetes (10)
21–23	Hypertension (3)
24–25	Asthma (2 practices)
26	Prescribing of benzodiazepines
27–28	Hysterectomy and hormone replacement therapy (2)
29–30	Vitamin B_{12} (2)
31	Thyroid disease
32	Oral contraceptive care
33–34	Lithium therapy (2)
35	Inadequate smears
36	Treatment of urinary tract infections in women of reproductive age
37	Topical steroids

2. Administrative

11–20	Appointments system (10)

38	Effectiveness of well person clinic
39	School leaving immunization
40	Health screening of the over-75s
41	Practice formulary
42	Patient satisfaction
43–44	Treatment room activity
45	Diet clinic
46	Outpatient referrals (counted as two audits)
47	Child surveillance
48	Use of x-rays
49	Appointment system for nurses' time
50–51	New patient registrations (2)
52–53	Recording of smoking and alcohol data
54	Prescription requests
55	Rubella immunity
56	Workload of a partner
57	Practice staffing strategy
58	Health promotion clinics

APPENDIX 6

Results of the conventional audits

The results of the conventional audits undertaken in 10 practices (5 in Lincolnshire and 5 in Manchester) are given below:

1. THE AUDITS OF DIABETES MELLITUS

Audit 1

A random 20 out of 50 identified non-insulin diabetic patients under 70 years were studied for the following parameters:

1. Seen in last 12 months? 100%
2. HbA1 in last 13 months? 100%
3. Weight in last 2 years? 50%
4. Blood pressure in past 2 years? 100%
5. Smoking history—ever recorded? 50%
6. Chiropody advice—any record? Not done in majority
7. Urine protein in last 2 years? Not done in majority
8. Lipids measured under aged 60 years? Not done in majority

Discussion: The question asked by the partners was: were the patients not asked or were the results not being recorded?

Decision: A rubber stamp was to be designed and inserted in the notes for a calendar year check by doctors. This protocol was to be applied to all diabetic patients including those seen at hospital clinics.

Audit 2

The audit population was randomly selected from the list of known diabetics and included 27 insulin dependent, 31 on oral hypoglycaemics, and 4 on diet alone—a total of 62 patients. The records were examined for the following parameters:

1. Seen in the past 12 months, and by whom? 91.9%, 88.7% by the general practitioner
2. Hospital follow-up? 66.7%
3. Weight recorded in last 12 months? 30.7%
4. Fundoscopy/eye check in past 12 months? 48.4%
5. Cholesterol level in the past 2 years? 11.3%
6. HbA1 in last 12 months? 33.9%
7. Monitoring of diabetes? Blood sugars 55.2%; urines 24.2%; no record 22.6%

Discussion: The results of the audit.

Decision: It was decided that the computer diabetic register should be updated regularly, and the medical record cover should be marked with a 'Diabetic' stamp. The continuation cards would be stamped with a list of the contents of the annual check, and particular emphasis would be placed on the 2-yearly cholesterol check. A further audit would be undertaken in 1 year.

Audit 3

This practice decided to audit against the following standards:

1. To provide enough care to prevent or detect treatable complications of diabetes.
2. To run a diabetic clinic and invite all known diabetic patients to attend by 1993.

3. All measurements and checks to be repeated at least annually.
4. To repeat audit in one year's time to evaluate the addition of a diabetic clinic.

The protocol used was to identify all known diabetics on the practice list (50), to re-assess the present standard of care and to offer better care and improve service to patients. All 50 diabetic patients were studied for the following parameters:

Patient details: Age, sex, treatment
Measurements: Weight 58%; blood sugar 58%; HbA1 44%; Urea and electrolytes (U & E) 14%; urinary protein 46%; blood pressure 64%; fundi 40%; pulses 22%; lipids 6%

Discussion: The partners felt they had not achieved the standards set and that a re-audit should show a significant upward trend in the measurement and recording of diabetic care and control following the start of the diabetic clinic and closer monitoring.

Decision: To re-audit in 12 months' time with all measurements; checks to be repeated annually with realistic targets set; and to invite all known diabetic patients to attend the clinic by 1993.
Targets to be:

1. Weight, blood pressure, urinalysis for protein, fundi, feet, blood sugar: 90%
2. HbA1: 60%
3. Lipids: 50%
4. U & E: 40%

Audit 4

A random selection of the notes of 20 diabetic patients of all treatment groups were examined for the following data recorded in the previous 12 months:

1. Weight? 30%
2. Blood pressure? 85%
3. Fundoscopy? 70%
4. Feet? 55%
5. Random blood sugar? 75%
6. HbA1? 30%
7. Urinary protein? 25%
8. Cholesterol? 10%

Discussion: Most of the patients attend hospital diabetic clinics, and it was felt that the level of recording in the general practice records was satisfactory, except for cholesterol levels. Omissions in the data were felt to be due to poor recording rather than failure to undertake the procedure. The discussion focused particularly on the care of elderly diabetic patients.

Decision: No further action was required at present.

Audit 5

The objectives of this practice were: "To get a good standard of care whereby patients and doctor are satisfied and good diabetic control is achieved, thereby hopefully minimizing the harmful sequelae and enabling the patient to maintain good quality of life."

It was decided to look at the care of 50 randomly chosen non-insulin dependent diabetic patients: 25 men and 25 women. The parameters chosen were:

1. All diabetic patients on oral hypoglycaemics should be reviewed by their general practitioner at least once every six months (go back three years).
2. The patient's blood pressure should be taken and recorded at least once a year (go back one year).
3. The patient should have fundoscopy performed annually and result recorded (go back one year).

Results were as follows:

	Men	Women	Total
Review (3 years)	24	24	96%
Blood pressure (1 year)	22	24	92%
Fundoscopy (1 year)	22	15	74%

Discussion: The doctors were pleased with the results and said the audit had been set deliberately at a low key to begin with and that they would re-audit in a more exacting form in one year.

Decision: Further investigations were to be undertaken regarding visual acuity recording, further discussion on methodology for fundoscopy, and recording of blood pressures was to continue to be reviewed annually.

Audit 6

This practice set out with the intention of assessing the level of metabolic control in its diabetic patients. The computer files of all diabetic patients were examined for the following:

1. Blood sugar in past year? 72%
2. Seen a general practitioner in past year? 92%

Discussion: An initial search of the computer diagnostic register yielded 50 patients, and the final total of 88 was derived using the prescription files.

Decision: It was decided that the doctors should write and follow a protocol for recording and caring for diabetic patients, and the 27 patients without blood sugar estimations in the past year should be followed up.

Audit 7

The protocol used by this practice for auditing their diabetic patients (insulin, tablets, diet) involved taking alternate notes at random from a computer printout of 88, 47 patients being studied altogether.

The following parameters and standards set were as follows:

1. HbA1—18 monthly? 80%
2. U & E—at least 5 yearly? 72%
3. Weight—at least annually? 72%
4. Blood pressure—at least annually? 93%
5. Risk factors: smoking/family history of cardiovascular problems—recorded? 51% and 21%
6. Pulses/feet—at least 2 yearly by doctor or nurse? 19%
7. Eyes—2 yearly by doctor or optician? 55%
8. Random blood sugar (RBS)—in last 3 years? 64%

Discussion: The results were considered to be fairly good but some of the problems encountered were:

1. Some notes were not legible
2. Inadequate hospital reporting from clinic visits
3. Summary sheets were not always up to date.

Decisions: These were:

1. To collect all information together and hold practice meeting regarding setting up of diabetic clinic by November 1992
2. To see all diabetic patients at practice clinic alternating with hospital clinic where applicable
3. To re-audit
4. To look at possibility of setting up separate eye clinic
5. To revise original protocol for diabetic care.

Audit 8

This practice set out to audit the attendances of all their diabetic patients (n = 96).

1. Seen general practitioner in past year? 65%
2. Seen at hospital in past year? 16%
3. Seen for other illness? 7%
4. Private patients? 5%
5. New patient? 1%
6. No follow-up at all in past year? 5%

Discussion: The results of the audit.

Decision: Although 93% of the patients had had contact with medical services, a decision was made to follow up non-attenders.

Audit 9

This practice undertook an audit of their diabetic care but they felt unable to share the findings with the project team.

Audit 10

The practice identified all known diabetic patients in order to assess the present standard of care with a view to offering better care through the newly set up practice diabetic clinic. Thirty-eight diabetic patients were studied (20 male and 18 female) (50%).

The following parameters were studied and results recorded:

1. Initial RBS? 53%
2. HbA1 in past 12 months? 58% (a further 30% had no record but possibly attended hospital clinic)
3. U & E in past 12 months? 42%
4. Lipids in past 12 months? 33%
5. Urinalysis in past 12 months? 61%
6. Testing own urine? 56%
7. Testing own blood? 42%
8. Weight in past 12 months? 53%
9. Blood pressure in past 12 months? 61%
10. Foot pulses in past 12 months? 22%
11. Chiropody attended? 50%
12. Fundoscopy in past 12 months? 69%
13. Referred to ophthalmologist? 28%
14. Evidence of neuropathy? 25%
15. Seen in hospital clinic in last year? 23; 1 private
16. Seen in practice clinic (running 1 year)? 67%
17. Seen by general practitioner in last year? 92%

Discussion: The main shortfall in the data was the absence of details on those patients attending the hospital clinic. Whilst the partners felt that these tests had probably been carried out, other practice staff reported that some patients had indicated that this was not always the case.

Decision: To design a rubber stamp with relevant boxes for use in notes as reminder of annual checks at the practice diabetic clinic (which increasing numbers of 'hospital' patients were choosing to attend).

2. THE AUDITS OF APPOINTMENT SYSTEMS

Audit 11

This practice looked at satisfaction of patients with the appointment system. Fifty patients were randomly chosen and questioned by the practice manager who recorded the answers on a tick chart. The questions asked were:

1. Did you obtain an appointment on the day you wished?
2. Did you specify which doctor you wished to see and was your preference arranged?
3. How satisfactory do you consider the appointment system to be?
4. Please advise what improvements you would like to see.

The audit found that only 12% had not been seen on the day requested; 10% were seen the next day; and 1 patient at another appointment of his choice. Of the 12% (6 patients), only 1 was angry but when asked for suggestions for improvements had none to offer. None of the 50 patients questioned offered any suggestions for improvement and everyone was satisfied with the system.

Discussion: Politeness bias was considered but not thought to be a relevant factor. The conclusions were that patients were generally well satisfied and were able to see the doctor of their choice at an acceptable time with all genuine emergencies seen the same day.

Decision: Whilst the practice would continue to give thought to improving the service, it was not felt that any immediate change was warranted.

Audit 12

This practice set a protocol for the appointment system audit and standards set were as follows:

1. All patients requesting an urgent appointment to be seen that day—target 100%
2. Patients who request to see the doctor of their choice should be able to do so within 3 days—target 80%
3. Patient should be satisfied with the appointment offered and service offered by reception when making appointment—target 90%

Data were collected by reception staff over a two-week period with all appointment requests recorded other than repeat bookings. The results were as follows:

Total appointments requested—393

(a) Emergencies? 14% (100% seen same day)
(b) Requested next available appointment (any Dr)? 41%
(c) Preferred named doctor (won't wait)? 2%
(d) Preferred named doctor (will wait)? 35% (89% seen in 3 days)
(e) Restricted by times? 6%
(f) Re-booking follow-up? 1%

Patient satisfaction was measured by a questionnaire given to 15% of patients attending an appointment during the two weeks of the audit. This was issued at random and replies were confidential.

1. Telephone: All answered 'yes' to getting through quickly.
2. Appointments: overwhelming majority considered a wait acceptable. Patients satisfied with time between request and appointment offered—97%
3. Patients' urgent appointments seen same day—100%
4. Patients who preferred to wait for choice of doctor but seen within 3 days—79.5%
5. Satisfaction with reception—majority said 'excellent'.
6. Surgery times—majority happy with existing arrangements.

Discussion: The partners were extremely pleased with the results of this audit.

Decision: No further action was needed at this time.

Audit 13

Questionnaires were given to all patients attending the surgery over 2 days, of which 116 were returned. The following were the key results:

1. 30% of patients considered their problem urgent.
2. 90% of patients were satisfied with the appointment given.
3. 29% were seen on the day of appointment request; 31% next day; 16% within 2 days; 25% 3 days or longer.
4. 90% said there was no difficulty contacting the surgery by telephone.
5. 60% waited less than 10 minutes after their appointment time; 30% 10–20 minutes; 10% over 20 minutes.
6. 10% spent under 2 minutes with the doctor or nurse; 35% 2–5 minutes; 40% over 5 minutes.
7. 80% felt that the appointments system was satisfactory.
8. 75% reported that the practice staff were 'helpful'.

Discussion: The 5-minute appointment system was felt to be contributing to the over-running of surgeries. The practice staff expressed much less satisfaction with the appointments system than the patients, and it was felt that there was room for improvement.

Decision: A re-audit was agreed, and the questions to be asked were refined.

Audit 14

A 2-day audit was undertaken with questionnaires for staff and patients.

1. 65% of patients were seen on the same day as their request; 21% waited one day; and 15% waited 2 days.
2. 92% saw the doctor of their choice.
3. 75% waited less than 10 minutes after their appointment time; and the remaining 25% waited less than 30 minutes.
4. At the beginning of surgery, 23% of appointments are still vacant.

Discussion: Most patients see the doctor of their choice within 2 days, and the majority are seen within 10 minutes of their appointment time and are satisfied with the system. Extra appointments are required, especially mid-week. This will require more room.

Decision: The appointment system will be continuously monitored.

Audit 15

This practice chose to look at doctor consultations for one year and telephone appointments. The aims were to:

1. Assess the consultation rate compared with the national average and to discuss the results.

2. Assess the accurate requirements of telephone lines and reflect peak periods for work-flow purposes.

The consultation audit was undertaken with the use of the practice computer and the telephone audit was completed by reception staff on a one-tick-per-call basis completed over a full working week.

The results showed that the practice conducted 41 327 consultations in 1991 averaging 3444 per month (492 per doctor per month or 25 individual doctor consultations per day). Peak consultation periods were January and July. The practice consultation rate of 2.9 per patient is below the national average of 3.5. The telephone audit revealed a total of 565 appointment calls over a 5-day period. Morning calls averaged 78 (Monday being the busiest with 144). Afternoon averaged 35 calls (Monday 51 calls).

Discussion: The conclusions reached were that:

1. The existing policy of 10-minute consultations may need to be revised if the practice seeks to improve its consultation rate and if there is patient demand for more availability. National consultation rates are based on 5/6 minute consultations.

2. The number of telephone lines estimated is sufficient but another line may be necessary if the list significantly increases, with the possibility of educating patients to telephone after 11 a.m. for test results.

It was felt that the conclusions of the telephone audit were correct but that, as only one Monday was included, the sample was too small.

The consultation rate figures give useful information for planning future surgeries but the mass of figures produced could not be accurately interpreted and possibly the consultation figures could be recorded on a weekly basis and graphed per doctor available to give a truer picture.

Decision: It was decided to re-audit on an annual basis.

Audit 16

The aim of this audit was to "assess the provision of appointments and to examine how well the practice is meeting the patients' requirements". The data for a complete year were used with the following findings:

1. 13 064 patients seen by the partners, 2258 by the trainee, 607 by locums.

2. 836 patients were seen in emergency appointments, 2766 at visits.

3. The consultation rate was 3.51 per patient per year (3.13 of which were in surgery).

Discussion: The appointments system was felt to be operating well except in August when there were fewer doctors present.

Decision: It was decided to reduce the clinics and increase the regular appointments in August. An imbalance of provision in emergency appointments—too many in the morning and too few in the afternoon—was recognized, and a shift in emergency appointments was agreed.

Audit 17

The practice set the following protocol when auditing the appointment system:

1. Patient satisfaction with the recently introduced five-minute appointments. (These five-minute appointments were added on to the lists of those doctors who were not on call for the day at the end of each evening surgery and were a continuous block of 6 five-minute appointments.)

2. Possibility of extending the five-minute appointments to morning surgery.

3. Time of day patients would prefer surgeries to be held.

The data were recorded on a simple questionnaire handed out to 50 patients at random over a two-day period:

1. Over previous 3 months, have you used a short appointment slot? 42% had; 58% had not.

2. If yes, did you experience any particular problems with:

   (a) Timing of appointment? Nil
   (b) Booking appointment? Nil
   (c) Waiting too long in waiting room? 14%
   (d) Was there sufficient time to satisfy your need? 44% yes; 4% no

3. Similar short appointment slots during morning surgery? 84% yes; nil no

4. Asked which surgeries they would like to see offered assuming surgery continues between 8.30 a.m. and 10.30 a.m.:

10.00 a.m.–11.00 a.m.	48%
11.00 a.m.–12.00 p.m.	8%
12.00 p.m.– 1.00 p.m.	26%
1.00 p.m.– 2.00 p.m.	10%
2.00 p.m.– 3.00 p.m.	32%
3.00 p.m.– 4.00 p.m.	4%
4.00 p.m.– 5.00 p.m.	30%
5.00 p.m.– 6.00 p.m.	14%
6.00 p.m.– 7.00 p.m.	64%

5. Happy to see a trained nurse for simple reviews rather than a doctor? 80% yes; 14% no

6. Lunch-time surgeries convenient? 62% yes; 34% no

Discussion: The results demonstrated that the 5-minute slots were appropriate when used properly and that a 6.00 p.m.–7.00 p.m. surgery would be popular. Extra information would be needed, however, owing to the extra costs involved, about who would use it and for what reason earlier surgeries were inappropriate. It was felt that the audit highlighted patients' ignorance of services offered and that this could possibly be the subject of a future audit.

Decision: It was decided that no changes would be made to the system until further information was to hand about the age and sex of people using surgeries and that, as this was perceived to be an ongoing problem, it would be re-assessed in one year.

Audit 18

This audit was undertaken on every 10th patient over a 6-week period (n = 315). The protocol, standards used, and results for the appointment audit were:

1. Length of waiting time for appointment—within 24 hours? 85%

2. Length of time in waiting room—within 20 minutes? 64.5%

3. Length of consultation time with doctor:

   0–5 minutes 46%
   5–10 minutes 39%
   10–15 minutes 13%
   15–20 minutes 1%
   20+ minutes 1%

4. Number of spare appointments as against extra patients seen in one week:

Spare appointments not taken up: total 65
Extra patients seen: total 68

Discussion: The partners were satisfied with the results shown.

Decision: It was decided to make no changes other than to keep the last two appointments free on Tuesday morning for emergency bookings that day.

Audit 19

Two hundred questionnaires were issued over one week between two centres, with 187 returned. The following questions were asked of the patients with the given results:

1. On making your appointment, did you consider your problem to be urgent or non-urgent? 37% considered it to be urgent; 63% non-urgent

2. Problems using telephone? 34% yes; 66% no

3. Appointment satisfaction 94% yes; 6% no

4. Wait to see doctor?

None	7.5%
Less than 5 minutes	16%
5–10 minutes	26%
10–20 minutes	35.5%
20–30 minutes	15%

5. Appointment of choice?

1st	78%

6. Time spent with doctor?

Less than 2 minutes	9%
2–5 minutes	38%
5–10 minutes	35%
10–20 minutes	15%
20–30 minutes	3%

7. Appointment system opinion?

Very poor	1%
Poor	3%
Average	31%
Satisfied	35%
Very satisfied	30%

Discussion: This initially focused around the telephone system. Deficiencies in the questionnaire and the need for objective measures of waiting time were discussed. The idea of involving patients in advising the practice was floated. Overall the practice felt that the appointment system was functioning satisfactorily.

Decision: It was decided to monitor appointment availability for Monday mornings and to measure the actual time that patients waited.

Audit 20

An audit was undertaken over four spring months to examine the distribution of appointments—some surgeries were under-booked and others over-booked. For each consulting session the number of spare appointments and extra patients seen were totalled.

The overall trends of appointment availability are as follows:

1. When no doctor was on holiday and there was a retainer doctor for two sessions on a Friday, there were surplus surgery appointments on every day of the week.

2. The above surplus appointments were more marked in the mornings than afternoons, at the greatest on Wednesday and Friday mornings, and at the lowest on Monday mornings.

3. There was normally a modest number of free appointments in the afternoons, except Friday when there were up to 55 free appointments.

4. During the months of April/May with one doctor away, there was a very close balance of appointments in the mornings Monday to Thursday with slight excess on Friday. There was a significant number of extra patients seen Monday, Tuesday and Wednesday afternoons over this two-month period.

Discussion: The dramatic effect of one doctor's absence on appointment availability was discussed. Morning surgeries had more availability than the afternoon ones, especially Tuesday.

Decision: Changes were agreed to the distribution of consulting sessions.

3. CLINICAL AUDITS

Audits 21 to 23

Three practices looked at *hypertension.*

One practice demonstrated that 35 (6.4% of the practice population) were being treated for hypertension.

Discussion: The frequency of blood pressure readings (average four a year) was regarded as satisfactory. However, the practice agreed the frequency of urine checks (15/35 within the past year) and urea and electrolyte estimations (20/35 within the past year) were unsatisfactory.

Decision: To institute a call-up system on the computer.

At a second practice:

Discussion: Whilst blood pressure checks were satisfactory (19/20 recorded in the last 8 months), the partners, as in the first practice, felt that the other unsatisfactory results highlighted the need for a new protocol to be written and instituted.

Decision: To write new protocol.

In the third practice, 20 patients with *hypertension* were audited.

Discussion: 19 out of 20 patients had a blood pressure recorded in the past 6 months, and half had a chest x-ray result in the notes; 9 (45%) had a full blood count recorded at diagnosis; 5 (25%) had had their fundoscopy recorded.

Decision: The practice protocol to be reviewed and amended to include the requirement for yearly electrolytes and urea in patients treated with thiazides and on patients with stable hypertension on beta blockers. It was agreed that younger newly diagnosed patients were to have their cholesterol measured and followed up if necessary. A chest x-ray and fundoscopy would be done on newly diagnosed patients as a baseline investigation. Hypertensive stickers would be put on notes and patients' compliance with monitoring would be checked through the prescription recall system.

Audits 24 and 25

Two practices undertook an audit of *asthma.*

One practice showed poor recording of data.

Discussion: Absent negative facts. For example, they were unsure whether an absence of a recording concerning a family history of asthma inferred that there was no family history or that the question had not been asked. Similarly, an absence of recording of inhaler technique might infer good technique or that it was not measured. (This issue arose in many audits and proved to be a major weakness in the use of medical records to gather audit data.)

Decision: The practice decided to write a new protocol and design a stamp as a reminder in the notes for improved recording. This was linked to the decision to increase the input from the practice nurses when seeing patients prior to the consultation with the doctor, both to record information and to improve patient education—which included assessing inhaler technique.

The second practice to audit asthma also showed the need to record more detail in the notes.

Discussion: They found in a sample of 26 of their 91 asthmatics that the peak flow rate had been recorded, at any time, in 69%, while 62% had been reviewed within the last year (58% within the last six months). That 15% of asthmatics were also smokers was felt to highlight the need for more effective patient education.

Decision: It was proposed that an asthma clinic be set up.

Audit 26

The *prescribing of benzodiazepines* was looked at by one practice to review the present system for repeat prescribing. This followed a previous review in 1988.

Discussion: The study audit showed that most men taking benzodiazepines were in the 50–59 age group and most women were in the 70–79 age group. Of 99 patients identified, 87 had been receiving treatment for three years or more with the majority having been reviewed three years ago or longer (73% were not reviewed annually). Despite the practice receiving no complaints about inappropriate prescribing, many of these patients had presented with falls and confusion.

Decision: It was decided that there should be more regular reviews and the review consultation should be recorded. A message would be printed on all repeat prescriptions of these drugs advising annual review and, after twelve repeats, a message to say a review was essential before further prescriptions would be issued. A re-audit would be undertaken in 12 months.

Audits 27 and 28

An audit on *hysterectomy and hormone replacement therapy (HRT)*, undertaken by a practice manager and senior receptionist, aimed to discover how many women on the practice list had had a hysterectomy with ovarian conservation; whether they had received advice on HRT; whether HRT had been prescribed; and whether they were presently taking HRT. Of 1027 patients within the cytology target age group, 67 were found to be excluded from the target owing to hysterectomy (6.5%). Among the 32 patients with a hysterectomy aged over 55, 14 (44%) did not appear to have discussed the possibility of HRT with a doctor or nurse in the practice. In the under-55 age group, 20 out of 35 patients (57%) equally had not had a discussion about HRT, and of these 80% had at least one ovary conserved.

Discussion: At the practice audit meeting, discussion centred on the use of HRT in patients with a history of carcinoma, the role of the practice nurse in preliminary discussions with patients, and HRT follow up in a clinic.

Decision: It was decided to write a letter to all patients aged under 55 who had had a hysterectomy, with or without ovary conserved, over the following 6 months and for all future hysterectomy patients to be sent an appointment for the HRT clinic within 6–12 months of operation.

Another practice undertook an audit on *hormone replacement therapy* since it perceived that there was a wide variation for monitoring of these patients. A computer search was made to identify all the women who had received a prescription for HRT over the period of a year—giving 83 patients. Of these 22 (27%) had been issued with repeat prescriptions; 70% of the women had had a smear and pelvic examination prior to starting HRT; and 85% had been examined within the subsequent 2 years; 90% of records had a blood pressure recording, and 80% had a breast examination.

Discussion and Decision: A protocol was written for the well woman clinic. Also it was agreed that new patients would have their past medical history checked, and smoking habits recorded. If the health check was satisfactory, the women for hormone replacement therapy will be directed to the well woman clinic for discussion and examination. The latter will include breast examination, and the recording of blood pressure and weight. Fasting serum lipids would be done if clinically indicated. The third decision was that a leaflet would be given to every woman already on hormone replacement therapy explaining the practice protocol, which would include six-monthly review.

Audits 29 and 30

Two practices undertook *vitamin B_{12} audits*.

One took 2 hours by a partner with the help of two clerks and an administration assistant. The aim was to review all patients on vitamin B_{12} and to provoke discussion among the partners concerning reasonable frequency of full blood counts (FBC). A computer search identified patients on hydroxocobalamin and a manual search of their clinical notes indicated the time of the last FBC; 95% of these patients had had an FBC within the past 2 years.

Discussion: This centred around the value of Schilling test in diagnosing pernicious anaemia; the ideal frequency of B_{12} injections; and the necessity for, and frequency of FBCs.

Decision: It was decided to continue treatment with existing patients already being treated with vitamin B_{12} but to look very carefully at new cases before instigating treatment.

Another audit of patients taking hydroxocobalamin was discussed in one practice. A flow chart for managing patients already receiving vitamin B_{12} injections was drawn up and discussed. Owing to the illness of the partner undertaking the audit, this audit was never completed.

Audit 31

An audit of the *treatment of thyroid disease* was done to facilitate the production of a protocol for the surveillance of thyroid function. This audit was undertaken in 2 hours by a partner and two clerks. A computer search identified all patients with diagnoses of myxoedema or hyperthyroidism, and those taking thyroid replacement therapy and/or anti-thyroid drugs. The clinical record was used to record the time of the last thyroid function test (TFT). Of 251 patients found, 20% were selected at random for analysis. All had received a thyroid function test within the last 15 months.

Discussion: The justification for annual testing was discussed and it was felt that often, if annual checks are consistently normal, five-yearly TFTs would be acceptable. An annual medication review was discussed, as was the need for a re-audit in one year.

Decision: It was decided to hold another meeting for further discussion on the emerging protocol.

Audit 32

An audit to look at *oral contraceptive care* was undertaken by a practice manager and completed in 6 hours. A list of patients receiving oral contraceptive care was identified and a random 1:5 selected (52 patients). The data recorded were:

Recorded within the past year:

Blood pressure?	86%
Weight?	63%
Smoking habits?	59%

Ever recorded:

History of jaundice?	28%
Family history (any diagnosis)?	26%
Epilepsy?	0.01%

Where recorded:

Yellow oral contraceptive cards?	69%
Notes?	17%
Not recorded?	13%

Accessibility of data:

Easily accessible?	69%

Discussion: The audit showed that some clinical points were infrequently recorded and the discussion focused on the need for a better designed recording card. The role of nurses in contraceptive care was also raised.

Decision: A re-audit was to be carried out one year after the new cards were brought into use.

Audits 33 and 34

One audit of patients on *lithium therapy* showed clear room for improvement.

Discussion: 79% of patients documented had lithium levels taken within the last year and this was felt to be satisfactory, but there were low levels of recording electrolytes and urea and thyroid function test results.

Decision: The practice set itself the target of three-monthly blood lithium level estimations and six-monthly renal and thyroid monitoring. As a result of this audit a card was placed in the medical records of all patients on lithium. On this card the doctor will record the serum lithium levels every three months, electrolytes, urea and thyroid function tests every six months. It was hoped that this would improve the standard of monitoring patients on lithium therapy. Another suggestion arising from this audit was an automatic recall system perhaps using the computer. This audit will be repeated at one year.

Another audit of *lithium treatment* was undertaken in one practice to establish the frequency of biochemical monitoring of patients on lithium, the focus of responsibility (hospital or general practice) for taking bloods, and to check on the system for receiving results and acting accordingly. Standards were set and seven patients receiving regular lithium carbonate were identified.

Standard agreed	Number of records meeting the standard (n=7)
Serum lithium to be taken 3 monthly	2
Blood for serum lithium should be taken 12 hours after last dose	1
Electrolytes and urea to be monitored annually	4
Thyroid function test to be done annually	5

Discussion: It was concluded that monitoring was haphazard and that lithium levels should always be known to the pre-scriber. There was much discussion about the responsibility of the practice when the hospital outpatients clinic takes blood tests within 12 hours of the last dose and does not pass on the result to the practice.

Decision: It was agreed that communication between the laboratory, hospital and practice should be reviewed, and the practice's computer record keeping improved. It was decided to re-audit in 12 months.

Audit 35

An audit undertaken to assess the percentage of *inadequate smears*, and the reason why they were inadequate, found that the results were better than expected.

Discussion: 3.5% of smears were reported as 'inadequate' compared to a 7% average for the district. This was confirmed by a regional treating centre.

Decision: Because there were no significant differences between the rates of inadequate smears taken by doctors or nurses, it was decided that patients requiring routine smears were to be referred to the practice nurses. It was also felt that it was reassuring to know that practice nurses could be relied upon to take smears properly, especially in the light of the pressure to meet targets.

Audit 36

An audit of the *treatment of urinary tract infections in women of reproductive age* aimed to assess differences in approach to the management of urine infections among the six doctors in the practice. It also aimed to investigate the use of urine culture before and after treatment and to identify the organisms involved; and finally, to identify the treatment given by each doctor.

Discussion: The results of the audit of 58 patients with urinary infection were as follows:

The culturing of urine:

No urine culture	21 (36%)
Culture before treatment started	36 (62%)
Of these: No growth	19
E. Coli	10
Coliforms	1
Proteus	1
No result available	4

Decision: The partners concluded that, since 83% of the positive urine cultures were due to *E. Coli*, it was reasonable to adopt a practice policy of prescribing trimethoprim when a urinary tract infection was suspected, without doing a pre-treatment midstream urine test. A urine culture would be done if the urine symptoms did not settle.

Audit 37

An audit of use of potent and very potent *topical steroids* revealed some interesting observations. The standards agreed by the practice were as follows. Patients should be seen each time a prescription was issued. A diagnosis should be made and recorded in the notes. Treatment should be started with mild or moderately potent steroids, as recommended in the *British National Formulary*. In all, 87 patients were identified of whom 26 patients had had two or more prescriptions. A diagnosis had been made in 18 (72%), no diagnosis had been made in 4 (16%), and in a further 3 the medical records were illegible; 9 (34%) of those receiving a repeat prescription had seen the doctor to receive it; 3 patients had been referred to a dermatologist.

Discussion: This audit led to discussion on the standard of record keeping in the practice and on the advisability of long-term use of potent topical steroid preparations.

Decision: No decision was made.

4. ADMINISTRATIVE AUDITS

Audit 38

An audit into the *effectiveness of the well person clinic* conducted by the practice nurse concentrated on the recording and management of weight.

Discussion: The practice felt that the results were acceptable, and justified the continuation of their diet clinic with only slight modification.

Decision: The practice decided to re-audit and to include blood pressure readings.

Audit 39

An audit to look at the *school leaving immunization* (diphtheria, tetanus and polio boosters) was done in one practice to ascertain the effectiveness of immunization on an opportunistic basis.

Discussion: The audit looked at a sample of 34 case notes of the 68 patients aged 17 and 18 and was undertaken by the practice nurses. This showed a 100% immunization uptake.

Decision: Despite this evidence of success, a regular call-up system has now been instituted and a small health check will be carried out at the same time as immunization since this was felt to be a better quality of service.

Audit 40

An audit looking into the *health screening of the over-75s* identified 319 such patients (7.4% of list). This was undertaken to ensure that the terms of service were being adhered to and to identify some of the problems encountered by the elderly. Of 76.5% who had been invited to have a health screening consultation, 80% asked for and had a home visit; 37.5% of assessed patients had significant problems identified.

Discussion: The practice was pleased that the audit confirmed that they were meeting their terms of service and that consultations appeared worthwhile in terms of identifying problems.

Decision: It was agreed to re-audit in 12 months.

Audit 41

One practice decided to look at their *practice formulary*, which had been introduced the previous year and which included 286 drugs, a total which excluded drugs usually initiated by hospital doctors. They wished to establish if the formulary was being adhered to (their standard was that 80% of prescriptions issued should be from the formulary) and to look at lessons learned for the formulary review when undertaken. Twelve *British National Formulary* (*BNF*) categories were checked, each taking about an hour, and the practice standard was met in nine.

Discussion: The results of the audit.

Decision: It was decided that all partners would attend a practice formulary meeting at which 24 drugs would be subjected to detailed discussion. It was also decided to re-audit in 12 months' time and encourage review on an annual basis.

Audit 42

In one practice an audit of *patient satisfaction* was conducted during morning surgeries over a two-week period including two busy Monday mornings. It was undertaken by the receptionists with the practice manager as co-ordinator and a partner as project manager. The aim of the audit was to evaluate patient reaction to various aspects of the morning appointment system and for doctors to gauge the system's effectiveness. A standard of 80% patient satisfaction was set.

Questionnaires were handed to all patients arriving for pre-booked morning appointments and 84% were returned. Of these, 92% had secured an appointment that day at their preferred time with 82% seeing the doctor of their choice; 91% were able to obtain an appointment when needed; and 73% were seen within 10 minutes of their appointment time.

Discussion: In the audit meeting the results were keenly discussed, in particular the difference in stress levels and waiting times following a previous change to 10-minute appointments. The practice also discussed the policy of seeing patients on the same day if necessary, staffing at busy periods, and the length of time telephones ring. The need for an audit of the number of calls for appointments during the first busy 3 hours in the morning and at other times of day was discussed, as was the need for improvements to the queuing system at the front desk.

Decision: It was agreed that patients were happy to wait up to 20 minutes after their appointment time provided they knew the reason for delay and a target was set as a future standard for auditing—everyone to be seen within 20 minutes of their appointment time.

Subsequent further discussions held by the practice manager with doctors and staff concluded that the result of the audit was satisfactory and, that whilst constantly under review, there was no requirement for a repeat audit earlier than one year.

Audits 43 and 44

Two practices decided to look at *treatment room activity*.

One practice wished to assess the frequency and type of use by casualties (urgent attenders), to compare the casualty frequency type seen between doctors and nurses and to look at the destination of casualties seen by nurses in the treatment room. This audit was undertaken over a two-week period but a breakdown in communication meant that only the practice nurse recorded data and not the doctors as specified. The results showed that less than 10% of casualties were seen and treated by nurses alone without seeing the doctor.

Discussion: This centred on the new facilities now available at the surgery and it was hoped to encourage patients to attend there rather than the nearest hospital casualty 12 miles away. This audit was not judged to be a success. This was partly due to the mix-up in data collection, but it was also clear that the audit did not address the practice's main question—was excessive time spent by the duty doctor in normal surgery time dealing with casualties? It was generally felt that it would have been more useful to have had a complete breakdown of nursing time spent on each task.

Decision: No decision.

In a second practice a small audit was conducted on the *treatment room workload for one month*. This showed that 142 bloods had been taken and 219 dressings done.

Discussion: The discussion centred on the time patients wait to have blood taken, which was sometimes up to a week.

Decision: It was decided to monitor the situation for a further month before reviewing the matter.

Audit 45

A *diet clinic audit* took the practice nurses in one practice about 12 hours. They did a questionnaire survey and gathered data from clinical records with the aim of assessing the clinical and practical effectiveness of the practice diet clinic. They were particularly interested in the feasibility of running a group clinic. The 50 questionnaires were unfortunately distributed to non-diet clinic attenders in error, resulting in only 18 replies. Of these 17 found the clinic helpful and 16 had lost weight; 15 indicated they would be interested in a group clinic. It was concluded that practice staff needed a clearer briefing before questionnaires were used and that the questions asked had to be more selective. However the result of 77% female and 73% male patients losing weight was a source of some satisfaction and patient feedback suggested that a group clinic was worth trying.

Discussion: The nurses expressed the need for more training in devising questionnaires and said they would give out questionnaires in the treatment room personally if a repeat audit was undertaken.

Decision: The practice decided to instigate two-monthly patient appointments in the clinic, with individual target weights and dates. Those patients unable to lose weight would be discharged.

Audit 46

An audit into *outpatient referrals* to consultants was carried out by a partner in one practice over a 10-week period. During this time 153 referral letters were written by the practice. They wished to ascertain whether patients had actually received an appointment from the hospital following a referral letter and the level of satisfaction with the appointment received.

A questionnaire was sent out to patients two weeks after the referral letter was sent and patients asked to return them within the following four weeks. Of the 98 replies received (69%) three had not received an appointment (they all eventually received one). Ten were discounted for various reasons (e.g. admitted to hospital before receiving appointment). A high level of dissatisfaction was expressed concerning appointments with ophthalmologists, orthopaedic surgeons and general surgeons but very little with ENT, obstetrics and gynaecology and physicians.

Discussion: This centred around the efficient use of the computer in audit, the results, and the difficulty of obtaining, in particular, orthopaedic appointments in under one year. They considered the possibility of offering an outpatients facility in the practice.

Decision: It was decided to send the audit results to the hospital, inform patients in the practice newsletter, and to re-assess the recording of data on the computer to increase their ability to audit referrals.

Audit 47

An audit of *child surveillance* in one practice was conducted by a partner with help from a health visitor and a receptionist. Notes were audited of 41 children aged between 4 years 3 months and 5 years. The general practice notes were not found to be as complete as clinic records and information was difficult to extract. The study, therefore, was based only on information available. The results were:

Standard	Audit against the standard	
All development checks should be completed within one month of stated times	6 weeks check	100%
	8 months check	100%
	18 months check	87%
	42 months check	63%

All children to be fully vaccinated by 4 years 3 months	Triple	100%
	MMR	95%
	Preschool boost	56%
Practice performing more than 50% of all vaccinations	Overall	31%
	Triple	39%
	MMR	51%
	Preschool boost	49%

Discussion: The standards of record keeping at the surgery and the difficulty in obtaining child care information from the district health authority. The health visitor felt very strongly that intensive visiting during the first year has great influence on future medical care.

Decision: It was decided that the health visitor would, in future, take the practice registration form for signing to birth visits at 14 days and give the patient an immunization record card to bring on visits to the surgery. It was also decided to bring forward the preschool booster recall letter to four years. The health visitor would begin reminding parents at $3\frac{1}{2}$ years about the 4-year check.

Audit 48

An audit was performed to identify all *x-rays ordered* over a two-month period. The data were collected by a partner. The number of x-rays performed was 48 (equivalent to 288 per annum at a rate of 54.3 per 1000 patients per annum). They were requested almost equally by each of the two partners and they had similar rates of detecting abnormalities (61% and 59% abnormal). Just over half the reports arrived between 15 and 21 days after a card was written. They considered the indications for x-ray, and the age and sex distribution of the patients.

Discussion: This centred around the results and, in particular, the length of time taken for the report to be received. The interval from request to report is principally the waiting period before the x-ray, rather than delay in issuing the report. The costings and reasons for x-ray requests were also discussed.

Decision: For the doctors to think carefully in future before requesting orthopaedic and spinal x-rays.

Audit 49

The *appointment system for nurses' time* was monitored in one practice for a month. The number of 5, 10, 15, and 20 minute nurse appointments was taken from the appointments book and other nursing activities were recorded and timed.

Discussion: The use of this information to justify the need for extra nurse hours to the family health services authority.

Decision: An agreement for the practice to employ an extra nurse.

Audits 50 and 51

New patient registrations provided the basis for audit in two practices.

One practice looked at all new patients registering over a three-month period and found that only 41% of registration medicals were undertaken, representing a loss of £2800 income on an annual basis.

The second practice set itself the target of examining 90% of all newly registered patients and claiming 100% of all possible fees. They examined 100 recent registrations and found that they had examined 63 of which 51 (81%) fees had been claimed.

Discussion: Both practices found that they were losing income as a result of patients not having a new patient health check, and both felt the need for receptionists to emphasize the benefits of new patient examinations on registration.

Decision: In one practice a procedure for new patient registration was drawn up and receptionists trained in its use. The other practice decided that if the initial invitation was disregarded, it was to be followed by a letter after two months. All invitations were to be recorded and checked. It was also decided to check retrospectively figures for numbers of registration medicals done by doctors and nurses, and check on forms that might be lost between the doctor and the administration. Both practices decided to re-audit at a later date.

Audits 52 and 53

Two simple audits on *the recording of smoking and alcohol data* were undertaken. Of 100 notes selected for the smoking audit, 48% had information on smoking and 12% were noted on summary sheets.

Discussion: This centred around the results of the audit, which were considered to be reasonably good. The practice has not yet done a re-audit but believes that heightened awareness about recording data has improved the quality of information recorded in notes.

Decision: To improve the quality of recording.

Of the 100 notes reviewed for the alcohol audit, 24% contained information, details or remarks about alcohol; 8% of these pertained to related problems or specific disease.

Discussion and Decision: A standard was devised to assign drinkers into light, moderate and heavy categories, making a uniform approach to classification on alcohol intake for all patients. Nurses were asked to record information on smoking and alcohol consumption at health checks.

Audit 54

The *number of prescription requests* that came into one practice was noted every day for two months providing the basis for a useful and interesting audit. The recording of 2260 repeat prescription requests occupied a quarter of the practice's staff time. The workload peaked on Mondays and Wednesdays.

Discussion and Decision: It was decided that, where appropriate, some patients could be changed from monthly to two-monthly prescriptions by doubling the amount prescribed. It was felt more logical if hypertensive patients were being seen every three months that their repeat prescriptions should be on a three-monthly basis. Finally it was agreed to encourage patients to come to the surgery or send for a prescription rather than use the telephone. This audit will be repeated to see if the new system is effective.

Audit 55

An audit of recording of *rubella immunity* in women of child-bearing age found that recording of rubella immunity did not meet the practice's agreed standard of over 80%. It was recorded in 34% of the medical records.

Discussion: It was suggested that rubella antibody testing should be offered to women requesting contraceptive services, undergoing fertility investigation, planning a pregnancy, attending for postnatal examination, attending for cervical smears, or newly registering at the practice.

Decision: A similar audit is to be undertaken in 12 months.

Audit 56

An audit of the *workload of a partner* was a consequence of the appointments audit.

Discussion: This audit cleared up a misunderstanding over the perceived workload of one of the partners, who believed he was doing more than his fair share of the work while others were doing less. He allocated one notional unit to each hour of consulting session, one unit to a day on call, one unit to an evening on call, and two units to a night on call. A weekend counted as 13 units and 3 visits counted as one unit, as did a meeting. He found that he was doing slightly less than he thought and that his partners were doing slightly more, and the workload of the partners closely mirrored their partnership shares. This helped to alleviate some disgruntled feeling and make for a better working atmosphere.

Decision: No decision was felt to be necessary.

Audit 57

An audit of the *practice staffing strategy* resulted, in the short term, in the termination of the contracts of two computer operators and a clerk being employed for $20\frac{1}{2}$ hours. The practice judged this audit to be very useful as it was the precursor to a longer term staffing policy which allowed planning time to train personnel to replace those leaving or retiring. It was also deemed to have saved the practice a considerable amount of expenditure.

Audit 58

Expenditure was also examined in an audit which looked at the potential and actual fees claimed for *health promotion clinics.*

Discussion: It was felt that a great deal of money was being lost because appointments at these clinics were not being taken up. The reasons for this were examined and it was found to be due to the loss of nurse cover.

Decision: It was decided to employ an extra nurse for health promotion clinic work.

COLLEGE PUBLICATIONS – EDUCATION

Vocational Training

The Future General Practitioner – Learning and Teaching
One of the RCGP's all-time best sellers. *'This stimulating and provocative book has been written by six outstanding general practitioners. It deserves to be read not only by teachers in general practice, but also by teachers in other fields of medicine'*
British Medical Journal £9.50 (£10.45 non-members)

A System of Training for General Practice (Occasional Paper 4)
This 'best seller' describes the philosophy of one department of general practice and outlines a practical method of organizing training for general practice. £7.50 (£8.25 non-members)

Clinical Knowledge and Education for General Practitioners (Occasional Paper 27)
Reports a study comparing the actions of groups of GPs and specialists faced with seven common clinical conditions. Useful for education and research in general practice.
£3.50 (£3.85 non-members)

Priority Objectives for General Practice Vocational Training (Occasional Paper 30)
The Oxford region's priority objectives for training: primary care, communication, organization, professional values and personal and professional growth. £3.50 (£3.85 non-members)

Course Organizers in General Practice (Occasional Paper 34)
This report of a major national survey of course organizers provides the most comprehensive and up-to-date information available on the subject. £4.50 (£4.95 non-members)

Towards a Curriculum for General Practice Training (Occasional Paper 44)
Examines several topical issues, including educational assessment, and does not shirk from tackling some of the major problems about current systems. £6.00 (£6.60 non-members)

A College Plan (Occasional Paper 49)
Comprises three statements approved by the Council of the College during 1989/90: An Academic Plan for General Practice, An Educational Strategy for General Practice for the 1990s, and The Faculties – the Future of the College.
£9.50 (£10.45 non-members)

Undergraduate Education

Undergraduate Medical Education in General Practice (Occasional Paper 28)
An AUTGP working group analyses the GMC recommendations on undergraduate medical education and the contribution which general practice can make. £3.50 (£3.85 non-members)

The Contribution of Academic General Practice to Undergraduate Medical Education (Occasional Paper 42)
The result of a questionnaire sent to all academic departments of general practice in the British Isles. Gives information on curricula, assessment procedures, staff training and teaching methods. £6.50 (£7.15 non-members)

Continuing Education

Continuing Education for General Practitioners (Occasional Paper 38)
Survey of the patterns of attendance at CME meetings comparing characteristics of GPs who attend regularly with those who attend occasionally or not at all. £5.00 (£5.50 non-members)

Higher Professional Education Courses in the United Kingdom (Occasional Paper 51)
A survey of 7 higher education courses with results and recommendations for future organizers. £6.50 (£7.15 non-members)

Portfolio-based Learning in General Practice (Occasional Paper 63)
A new approach to higher professional education based on a technique of personal learning. £9.00 (£9.90 non-members)

Assessment

What Sort of Doctor? (Report 23)
Describes the most radical system so far published on the assessment of performance review by GPs in their own practices.
£5.00 (£5.50 non-members)

Practice Assessment and Quality of Care (Occasional Paper 39)
An extensive review of the literature of assessment and quality in general practice with special reference to practice visiting.
£7.50 (£8.25 non-members)

Rating Scales for Vocational Training in General Practice (Occasional Paper 40)
A set of 23 rating scales, with subscales, from the Department of General Practice at Manchester enabling trainers to monitor progress of trainees during their general practice year.
£5.00 (£5.50 non-members)

Practice Activity Analysis (Occasional Paper 41)
Describes the results of practice activity analysis undertaken by the RCGP Birmingham Research Unit over a number of years and discusses its role as a practical approach to audit and assessment of quality. £7.50 (£8.25 non-members)

Examination for Membership of the Royal College of General Practitioners (MRCGP) (Occasional Paper 46)
A comprehensive overview of the MRCGP examination: its development, current state and future trends. Includes sample questions and answers. £6.50 (£7.15 non-members)

Fellowship by Assessment (Occasional Paper 50)
The latest quality assurance programme in general practice from the College based on research and peer review and giving the history of its development. £7.50 (£8.25 non-members)

Multidisciplinary Education

Education for Co-operation in Health and Social Work (Occasional Paper 14)
Reports an interdisciplinary conference of social workers, nurses, health visitors and GPs. £3.00 (£3.30 non-members)

Working Together – Learning Together (Occasional Paper 33)
This reports the successes and failures of courses run to promote teamwork in general practice. £3.00 (£3.30 non-members)